PREFACE

There are hundreds of textbooks devoted to Anatomy, Physiology, Biochemistry, Pathology, Medicine, and Surgery with tomes on their various specialities, such as my specialty of Orthopaedics, as well as Radiology and Haematology to name just a few. There is a book of 500 pages devoted to the front half of the foot! I have written this book as a guide to better understanding how doctors think and how you may understand their terminology, as well as a guide to problems within the musculo-skeletal system.

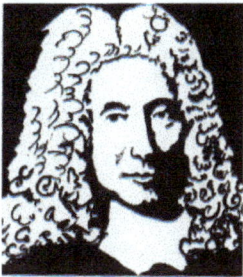

In 1741, **Nicolas Andry,** 1658-1742 made up the word "Orthopaedia" from two Greek words *Orthos* — straight — and *pais* — child — or *paedia* — the study of children, meaning "straight children" who, with splintage for legs bent from rickets, would grow straight like the tree tied to the stake. The image on the front cover is the orthopaedic tree. This tree has become the symbol of every Orthopaedic Society in the world. Orthopaedics has grown to include adults as well as children and embraces the musculo-skeletal system.

◆ Nicholas Andry

I have been greatly influenced by the late **Alan Graham Apley,** 1914-1996, who believed in simple English, was a superb teacher, a fine Orthopaedic surgeon, and author of a comprehensive textbook on Orthopaedics.

I dedicate this book to his memory.

CONTENTS

FOREWORD

We communicate by words. The meaning can be misinterpreted when one person says something, and the other person hears something else or misconstrues what is meant. This is particularly true when a consultation takes place between a doctor and a patient, especially if a word the doctor uses is from Latin or Greek. A person can believe a fracture is worse than a break when they both mean the same.

Sometimes a word is emotive, like cancer or whiplash, and when one hears the word cancer one fears death will follow, when it may be a benign or harmless growth, proving only half of what is said goes into your brain.

The internet does not always provide the best source of knowledge but is enormously helpful in finding out about certain conditions. The history of medicine is full of examples when an idea is not accepted because it is new and runs contrary to what is believed.

William Harvey, 1578-1657, found the circulation of the blood in 1625, but his colleagues had been taught from Galen's time (1500 years earlier) that the heart pumped the blood back and forth like the tides going in and out.

This picture shows Harvey demonstrating the flow of venous blood back to the heart and the back flow blocked by valves. They would not accept the new concept that blood was pumped around the body and back again. It seems laughable now, but not then. **Michael Severtus,** 1511-1553, was burnt at the stake in 1553 for suggesting the pulmonary circulation, as well as other heresy.

An idea such as washing one's hands to prevent carrying infection from one person to another took over a hundred years before it was accepted and, even then, the discovery of the microscopic organisms did not convince everyone.

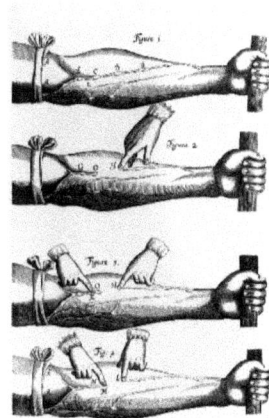

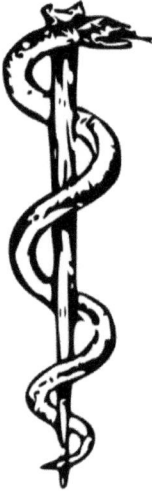

Asclepius was the ancient Greek God of healing and temples were built in his honour. His staff featured a rod with a snake twisted around it and this has become the symbol for doctors down the ages.

Hippocrates, ?460-375 BCE, (Before Common Era), built a hospital on Cos, and is considered to be the Father of Medicine. His students undertook an oath which is still used today in a modified form at the graduation ceremony following a course of study at Medical School. Basically, it is: "To do my best and do no harm."

The field of Orthopaedics has grown, but it is now splintering into subgroups with specialists in the upper limb, or even just the shoulder, elbow, or hand, and lower limb, with hip, knee, and ankle, and the spine. It will probably end with someone specialising in the big toe!

I would encourage readers to search out the persons listed in bold throughout the text as to their contributions to medicine. Much can be learnt from history even though it cannot be changed.

Notes:

WHAT WE ARE MADE OF

We are made of stardust; formed from the original supernova explosion which made the solar system, powered by our sun. We are a carbon-based animal. The following applies to other animals besides humans.

This is a eukaryotic cell from the beginning of life over three billion years ago and is still present today in all of our cells.

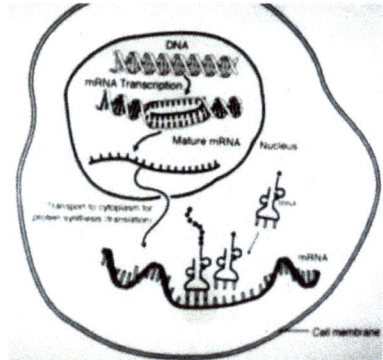

All the essentials of life are contained within the nucleus of cells in the form of chromosomes composed of DNA (De-oxy ribo-Nucleic Acid): a double-coiled helix of carbon atoms linked by short proteins called amino acids with adenine and guanine on one side, linked to thymine and cytosine on the other. Information is passed by Messenger Ribo Nucleic Acid (mRNA).

Each cell in our body contains 46 chromosomes.

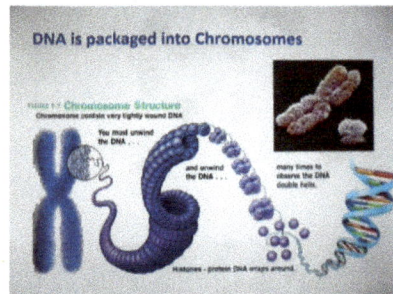

DNA is packaged into Chromosomes

The genetic material is known as genomes and is found on two of the 46 human chromosomes. XX for women and XY for men.

Each egg and sperm contain half the number of chromosomes and when combined the information is passed onto each daughter cell.

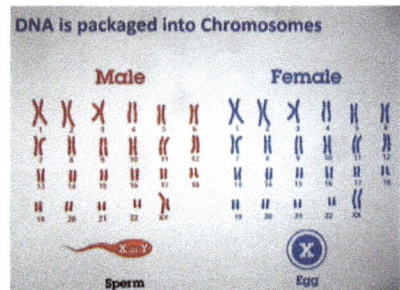

DNA is packaged into Chromosomes

Each of us is unique, unless a fertilised egg splits and identical twins or triplets are formed which are genetically the same. If two or more eggs are fertilised at the same time, separate individuals are formed, or non-identical twins.

When the DNA splits it is taken by mRNA to make another replica.

Notes:

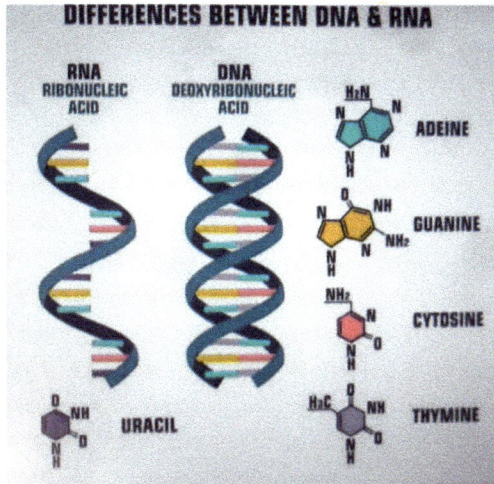

DIFFERENCES BETWEEN DNA & RNA

RNA RIBONUCLEIC ACID

DNA DEOXYRIBONUCLEIC ACID

ADEINE

GUANINE

CYTOSINE

THYMINE

URACIL

MALE GENETIC MATERIAL is carried in the sperm manufactured in the testes, located in the scrotum, outside the body as they need a slightly cooler temperature (3°< the core body temperature) to develop. They are miniscule, with a head containing the father's DNA and a mobile tail called a cilium (plural cilia), to enable it to swim.

They are stored in the epididymis, a densely coiled tube (6 metres in length if uncoiled) attached to the surface of the testis, which then links to the vas deferens (like a small hose) to the base of the bladder, where they are stored in the seminal vesicles, behind the prostate gland. Between 250-300 million are released at ejaculation, contained in about a teaspoon of creamy material from the prostate through an erect penis.

The penis is the conduit for the bladder via the urethra.

It is composed of erectile tissue, normally limp, but when a male is aroused, it fills with blood to become hard to enable entry to the vagina of a woman. If the male is uncircumcised the foreskin is retracted to expose the sensitive glans or head of the penis.

The testes also are endocrine (internal) glands secreting testosterone, responsible for the changes which occur at puberty with deepening of the voice, growth of hair on the face and at the pubic area, and an interest in the opposite sex (as a rule).

Notes:

FEMALE GENETIC MATERIAL is carried in an egg or ovum, (plural ova), manufactured in an ovary located on either side of the pelvis. Each ovary contains almost a million eggs at birth, but at puberty has only about 300. They are about the size of the head of a pin and contain the mother's DNA. They undergo a cycle within the ovary once a month when one matures (ovulation) and is expelled into the fallopian tubes (**Gabriele Fallopio**, 1523-1563) which are connected to the uterus (womb).

The uterus is a muscular (myometrium) organ, lined by a vascular lining (endometrium) connected to the vagina, (a hollow continuation of the female genital tract), at the cervix. The vagina opens through the muscular pelvic floor in front of the anus or terminal portion of the large bowel, and in front, the urethra, the tube through which urine is expelled from the bladder. The uterus accepts a fertilised egg, and, via a placenta (a vascular plate), matures this into a baby.

For a woman to become pregnant naturally, the erect engorged male penis enters the vagina and at climax, or orgasm, expels the teaspoon of semen containing millions of spermatozoa at the mouth of the uterus allowing them to swim upwards where one will meet an egg in the fallopian tube.

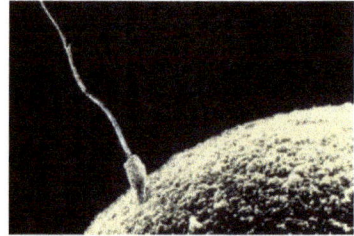

Note the size of the sperm with the egg.

Sometimes they meet outside, and an ectopic pregnancy can occur.

Artificial Insemination or Artificial Invitro Fertilisation (AIF), is a means where sperm are collected, stored, and implanted into an egg collected from a woman at ovulation.

The ovaries are also endocrine glands secreting the hormone oestrogen into the blood stream, which also changes a girl into a woman at puberty with enlargement of the breasts, widening of the pelvis, and the menarche or commencement of menstruation.

This occurs because the lining of the uterus is thickened with new blood vessels in case the egg is fertilised. If it is not, the oestrogen is cut down and the lining is shed which may take three to four days. It is called a period. It is a cycle lasting about a month with ovulation usually occurring in the middle.

If the egg is fertilised, another hormone, progesterone, is secreted which stops the shedding of the uterine lining.

If the woman misses one, she suspects she may be pregnant and is certain if she misses two. This can now be confirmed by a pregnancy test which measures the level of hormones in the urine. She may also have morning sickness, as she is nurturing a foreign person within her, with her and her partner's DNA mixed.

When a sperm and an egg (ovum) unite, they form a new organism, called a zygote, which starts to divide. Note the size of the sperm as it approaches the egg (previous page). Once it enters the egg, an enzyme (chemical) is secreted prohibiting entry to any other sperm. Each ovum contains an X and each sperm an X or Y. Therefore, there is an equal chance of the zygote becoming a boy or girl.

The cells divide initially into two and then again, doubling very quickly. The division of the zygote from the beginning into two halves is finally represented by the cleft in the upper lip seen on all humans and sometimes in the vertebrae on chance x-ray of the spine.

Within three to four days the multinucleated cell implants into the wall of the uterus and continues to grow.

Up to eight weeks the developing baby is called an embryo and after that a foetus. Stem cells divide into three basic tissues: ectoderm (the outer layer) which gives rise to the nervous system and the skin; endoderm (the inner layer) which gives rise to the alimentary canal, its lining, and the glandular structures that develop from it such as the liver and pancreas, also the respiratory and genitourinary system; and mesoderm (the middle layer) which gives rise to the muscles, bones, and joints or the musculoskeletal system.

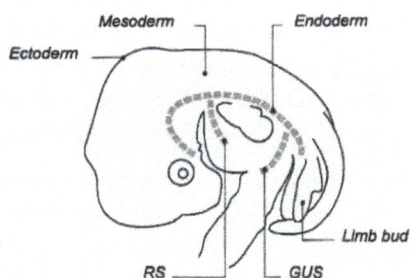

6 Week old Embryo

Nutrition from the mother develops via a placenta joined to the embryo by an umbilical cord. After eight weeks the embryo becomes a recognisable human foetus and spends the remaining time in the uterus until a viable age (now reduced to 24 weeks) arrives, although most babies need until 40 weeks or nine months, before they are sufficiently able to survive the cold, hard world outside the womb.

The body consists of many different sets of tissues, made up of individual cells with a similar function, called systems. They are all interdependent. The body weight consists of 60% fluid, 40% within the cells, and 20% extracellular.

Notes:

There are three different types of cells that make up the different systems:

LABILE

These are capable of reproduction and usually do reproduce all the time.

It is said that the whole skeleton is usually replaced within seven years as old bone is taken away and new bone is laid down (fortunately not all at once).

Cells are lost continuously from the skin surface, and from the lining of the gut and lungs. These cells are the ones that usually respond to extraneous stimuli to become malignant.

The suffix -blast is used to describe cell formation such as bone (osteo) forming cells (osteoblasts); -clast or -phage to describe cells that break down tissue (osteoclasts) or blood cells that ingest and break down tissue (macrophages); and -cyte to denote stable cells such as bone cells (osteocytes).

STABLE

These cells are only capable of reproduction when needed such as cells within the liver.

PERMANENT

These cells lack the ability to reproduce and damage to these cells is usually permanent. Nerve cells, muscle cells (myocytes), and cells forming the cartilage lining joints (chondrocytes) fall into this category.

Over time eventually all systems fail, and we die. However, the body is remarkable how it can withstand the various accidents and diseases we encounter. Life expectancy has been increasing over the past 100 years such that most humans can expect to reach their 80s, especially within the developed nations. This also raises problems of care and how to help an aging population cope.

All cells contain nuclei which release information from their DNA via mRNA (messenger RNA).

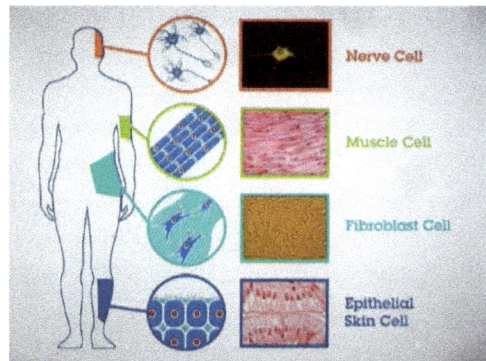

Picture courtesy of Dr J Philps.

Notes:

NS: NERVOUS SYSTEM

This is divided into CENTRAL and PERIPHERAL. The brain interprets all information.

We also experience emotions, and this could be called the PSYCHOLOGICAL system and is what we think about and experience. It is also under the influence of the various hormones excreted by the glands within the body (endocrine glands), such as the release of adrenaline when being chased by a bull for example, and which can also show from the exocrine glands which connect to the surface of the skin such as moist palms when in an exam.

It is influenced by parents, teachers, TV, religion, books, even diet, notwithstanding advertisers. Counsellors, Psychiatrists and Psychologists can help in times of stress.

There are inner senses related to this which my father **Sir John Walsh,** 1911-2003, taught me:

A sense of personal worth, or self-esteem. It is reinforced by our parents' belief in the worth of their child and is mainly contributed by the mother.

A sense of the worth of others, respect. Again, this is related to the parents' beliefs and also contributed by the attitude of the society in which we live. Jews were outcasts in Hitler's Germany in the 1930s to 40, such that a policy of genocide ensued, resulting in the Holocaust.

A sense of awe, wonder at the marvels around us such as a rainbow, a sunset, a flower, a painting or piece of music.

A sense of proportion, to know what is important and what takes priority.

A sense of humour, even to laugh at oneself.

The ability to communicate is by language, and we need to protect and preserve it. English has become the main language of communication. Tik Tok, Twitter and other social media do not always tell the truth.

CENTRAL NERVOUS SYSTEM

Although the brain and spinal cord receive a large proportion of blood (15-20%), the cells are bathed in cerebro-spinal fluid (CSF) produced by the choroid plexuses (a rich system of blood vessels) in the lateral, third and fourth ventricles, a system of cavities within the brain and brain stem. It is enclosed in three coatings called the meninges.

Notes:

The innermost is the pia mater adherent to the surface, the intermediate the arachnoid mater, and the outer and thickest the dura mater. The CSF is between the arachnoid and the pia forming a protective and nourishing fluid and the capillaries supplying the brain cells.

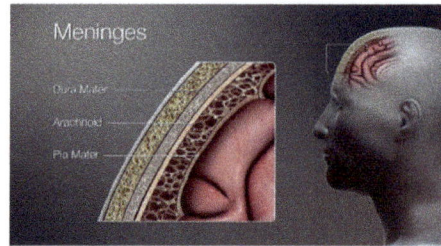

Central System (Brain):

This part is known as the cerebrum, cerebellum and brainstem.

The cerebrum is divided into two hemispheres connected by the corpus callosum, a thick bundle of nerve fibres. The left half controls the right side and the right the left.

Information entering the brain is known as the sensory system and information leaving is the motor system. There are about 100 billion cells (grey matter) in the brain linked by nerve fibres or axons (white matter) which are connected by synapses, allowing chemical transmitters to pass information.

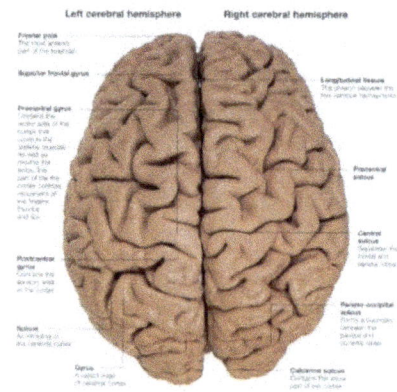

The cerebrum consists of the cortex folded to fit the space of the skull, with the folded-up part called the gyrus and the fold the sulcus. The base is known as the cerebellum and brainstem exiting through the base of the skull as the spinal cord. The cerebellum takes care of the functions we do not usually think about such as the heart beating, breathing, digestion, maintaining posture, and walking.

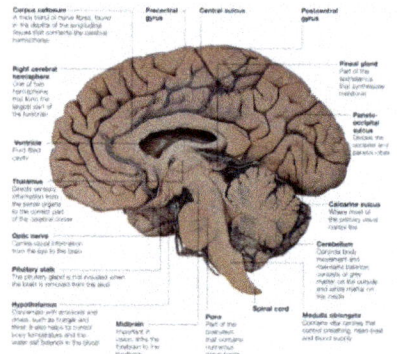

The brain itself has no sensation and this has allowed scientists to find the different areas of the brain that control information. The five major senses are: touch, sight, hearing, smell, and taste.

Notes:

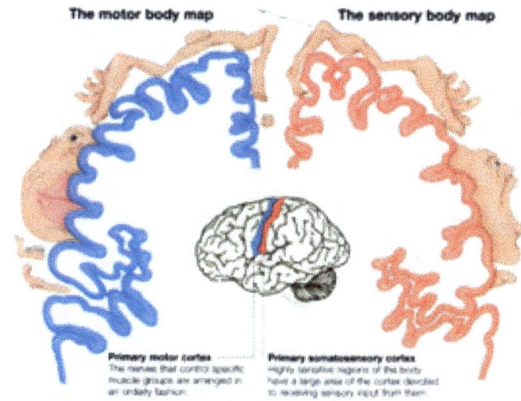

The motor body map   The sensory body map

Primary motor cortex
The nerves that control specific muscle groups are arranged in an orderly fashion.

Primary somatosensory cortex
Highly sensitive regions of the body have a large area of the cortex devoted to receiving sensory input from them.

TOUCH:

This is conveyed from sensory cells in the skin or other surfaces. Proprioception is similar in that the cells in moving joints can convey position sense. This area of the brain is located in front of the motor cortex which controls the skeletal muscles. The left half controls the right and vice versa with the fibres crossing in the corpus callosum. Note the homunculi denoting the amount of brain devoted to the face and hands.

SIGHT:

We have a camera eye where the cells sunk beneath the skin to form a retina, with an outer clear layer (cornea) with light modified by an expandable shutter (iris, blue or brown) and movement of the eyeball by muscles. A lens developed to focus the light on the retina which in humans consists of rods that see low levels of light but no colour, and cones which do see colour. The image is upside down optically but is processed into the correct position by the brain after receiving the images sent via the optic nerve.

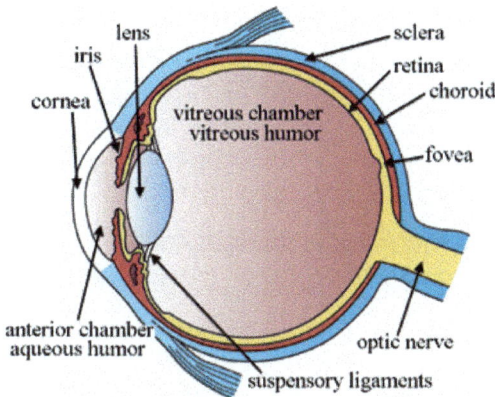

lens
iris
cornea
sclera
retina
choroid
vitreous chamber
vitreous humor
fovea
anterior chamber
aqueous humor
optic nerve
suspensory ligaments

Notes:

HEARING:

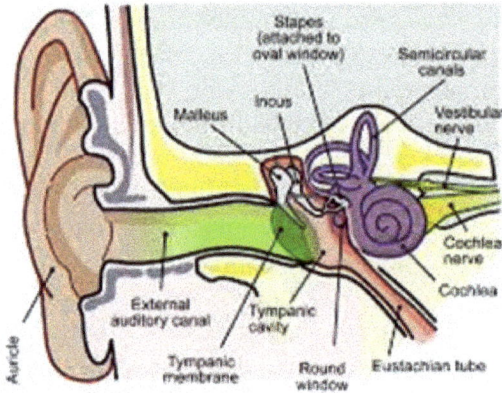

What we hear is sound. Sound is transmitted by a wave and needs a medium for the wave to travel such as water or air. Low frequency waves are low in pitch and high frequency shriller. The ear is located at the side of the head. There is the outer ear which we see, the middle ear, and the inner ear. These are separated by a thin stretch of membrane similar to a drum skin and naturally are called an ear drum or tympanic membrane.

There are three tiny bones in the middle ear, called the malleus (hammer), incus (anvil), and stapes (stirrup). They are the smallest bones in the human body and do not grow after birth. The malleus is attached to the outer membrane and the stirrup is attached to a smaller inner membrane (oval window). The eustachian (auditory) tube connects the middle ear with the nose to equalise the air pressure and this is commonly affected when flying in airplanes or diving. The inner ear contains the cochlea filled with fluid and tiny hairs connected to the auditory nerve.

Waves of sound push on the tympanic membrane, and this causes movement across the chain of bones to push on the oval window with movement in the cochlea enabling hearing.

The human hearing range is 20- 20Kilo-(20,000) Hertz (Hz). As one ages the higher frequencies are lost and you can often see older men cupping their hands behind their ears or just nodding and smiling, not having heard a word.

Modern hearing aids which fit in the ear and are powered by tiny batteries have helped them (the author included) tremendously. Deaf people can be very creative, and Beethoven composed his best works when he became completely deaf. Cochlea implants are now being used for the profoundly deaf.

Notes:

The organs of balance or semi-circular canals are also filled with fluid and give position sense to the head, similar to a gyroscope. These are affected by unusual motion, such as at sea in a small boat causing seasickness.

SMELL:
In humans there are multiple nerves in the roof of the nose which pass through what is called the cribriform plate to the brain in the form of the olfactory nerve. Molecules of scent cause impulses which are interpreted, from birth with the scent of the mother from breast feeding. The molecules in the air dissolve in the mucous membranes of the nose. Wine connoisseurs are even called "a nose"!

TASTE:
This is mediated by the tongue and soft palate with receptor cells located in the taste buds. There are five basic tastes with sweet, sour, salty, and bitter, and more recently umami discovered by the Japanese being the savory taste of free glutamates (e.g. mushrooms, cured meats, cheese, seaweed). These tastes can be enhanced by the addition of monosodium glutamate.

PERIPHERAL NERVOUS SYSTEM

This transmits impulses through the spinal cord to the brain. Nerve cells are located in the spinal cord and their axons transmit the impulses from the motor cortex to receptors in muscles, whilst end organs in the sensory system transmit impulses to the sensory cortex. Try walking in bare feet after a child has been using Lego.

They emerge sequentially from the spinal cord and sensory levels are known as dermatomes; see the image on the next page.

CVS: CARDIOVASCULAR SYSTEM

The heart is a muscle which pumps blood around the body and through the lungs for re-oxygenation. Blood consists of cells and plasma. There are around five litres of blood in an adult, of which two litres are cells and three litres are plasma.

Notes:

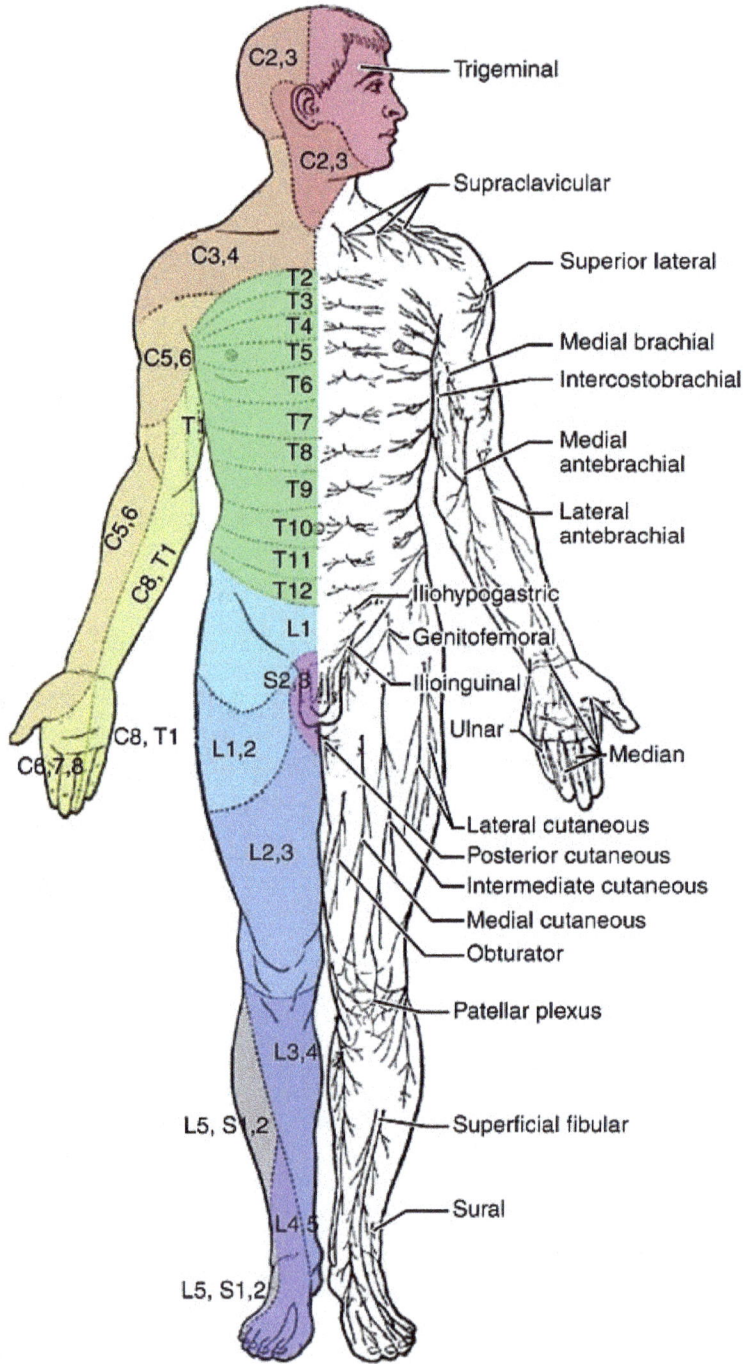

C2,3 — Trigeminal

C2,3

C3,4

Supraclavicular

Superior lateral

T2
T3
T4
T5
T6
T7
T8
T9
T10
T11
T12

C5,6

T1

Medial brachial

Intercostobrachial

Medial antebrachial

Lateral antebrachial

C5,6

C8,T1

Iliohypogastric

L1

Genitofemoral

S2,3

Ilioinguinal

Ulnar

C8, T1

C6,7,8

L1,2

Median

L2,3

Lateral cutaneous
Posterior cutaneous
Intermediate cutaneous
Medial cutaneous
Obturator

Patellar plexus

L3,4

L5, S1,2

Superficial fibular

L4,5

Sural

L5, S1,2

Above: Peripheral Nervous System

HS: HAEMO-POIETIC SYSTEM

(Pronounced heemopoyetik), this is where blood is made and unmade. The cells are manufactured in the bone marrow and spleen (an organ just under the left side of the diaphragm), the muscle separating the thorax (chest) and abdomen.

Red cells (erythrocytes), a biconcave disc containing haemoglobin, an iron-containing molecule, which carry oxygen; white cells (leucocytes and lymphocytes) which fight bacteria and viruses; and platelets, which help seal wounds and promote clotting. Red cells survive between three to four months and are broken down in the spleen and liver with the haemoglobin reused in the bone marrow to make new cells. The white cells last only one to two days and are regenerated in the spleen and bone marrow. Plasma is a watery, slightly yellow-coloured fluid which contains clotting factors, proteins, and nutrients.

CVS (CONTINUED)

There are two parts in the heart, separated by a muscular septum and each has a receiving chamber, called the atrium, and a discharging ventricle which acts as the main pump. They contract synchronously.

The flow is controlled by valves which are closed forcibly, and these are the sounds heard through the stethoscope and sound like lub, dupp. The rate is controlled by a nerve supply and also by hormones such as adrenaline.

The right half receives the de-oxygenated venous blood (blue) and pumps it to the lungs and the pulmonary veins bring the now oxygenated blood (red) to the left half which pumps it around the body and, as such, is bigger and stronger. The arterial system takes the blood from the heart and the venous system returns it.

There are valves in the peripheral veins which assist the flow back to the heart as they are thin walled as opposed to the thicker walled muscular arteries. When the valves fail in the legs varicose veins appear.

100% of the venous circulation enters the right half and leaves via the pulmonary arteries to the lungs where oxygen and carbon dioxide exchange takes place. This blood returns to the left half and is pumped through the body via the aorta and other arteries to the brain (20%), the alimentary system (20%), the kidneys (20%), the muscles and bones (20%), and the heart itself with the skin and endocrine glands (20%).

Notes:

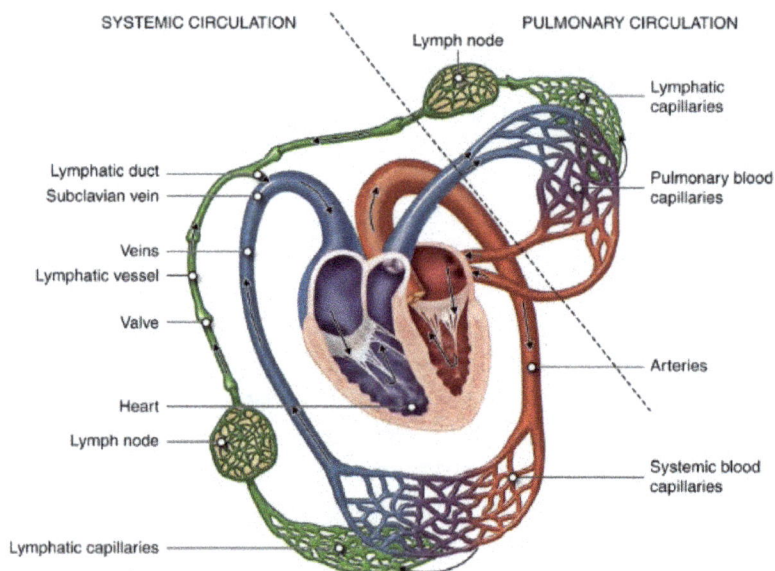

Above: Cardiovascular and Lymphatic System

Exercise increases demand and more blood is diverted to muscles.

Oxygen exchange is through the thin, tiny capillaries linking the two systems. These were discovered by **Marcello Malpighi,** 1628-1694, in Italy in 1661, years after Harvey had postulated them.

LS: LYMPHATIC SYSTEM

This consists of the tiny channels that bring fluids leaked from the blood vessels back into the blood vascular system, via nodes (often, wrongly, called glands) which filter bacteria, or neoplastic cells and can become inflamed and swollen. The lymph is returned to the venous system by the thoracic duct (refer to image above).

THE SKIN

This is made up of an outer layer of flattened (squamous) cells or epidermis, the dermis beneath and the subcutaneous layer beneath that. The exocrine glands producing sweat, hair follicles, nerve endings and blood vessels are contained in the dermis and subcutaneous layer, and give control to maintaining body temperature.

Notes:

RS: RESPIRATORY SYSTEM

This consists of tubular passages from the nose and mouth via the larynx and trachea, which you can feel in the front of the throat below the Adam's apple, bronchi, bronchioles to the alveoli (tiny sacs) where oxygen exchange takes place and CO_2 and water are excreted from the lungs. Air pressure drives the air in when the diaphragm and rib cage are expanded to create a partial vacuum and when relaxed, expel the air.

GUS: GENITO-URINARY SYSTEM

This consists of the kidneys, ureters (tubes) and bladder filtering waste products from the blood excreting them in the urine; and the reproductive organs. The urine is collected in the bladder and excretion is controlled by a muscular sphincter until a certain pressure triggers impulses to the brain to be emptied (if convenient), via the urethra.

AS: ALIMENTARY SYSTEM

This consists of the mouth and gut where food is ingested, ground up by the teeth, digested in the stomach and small intestine, absorbed and excreted. Enzymes (chemicals) secreted by the saliva in the mouth commence digestion, before the food is swallowed and passes to the stomach, via the oesophagus. It is retained for some hours and broken down by acids secreted by glands in the stomach wall. Mucus from adjacent glands prevent digestion of the stomach wall. The acid is neutralised by secretion from the pancreas and bile from the liver via the gall bladder, as it passes via the duodenum, a C-shaped loop into the small intestine, jejunum and ileum.

Further absorption occurs from the small projections in the wall called villi (singular villus). The broken-down chemicals enter the blood stream and are filtered through the liver before entering the heart and dispersal to the body in carbon fragments for use by the different organs of the body. The waste enters the large bowel at the caecum then the ascending, transverse, descending sigmoid colon, and is further modified before passage to the rectum and from the anus as faeces.

ES: ENDOCRINE SYSTEM

This is under the control of the pituitary gland located in the brain under the optic nerve chiasma, where they cross. This gland secretes hormones, (chemicals) directly into the blood stream and affects the different glands, otherwise known as ductless or endocrine glands, on their production of hormones in a feedback loop, which affect various metabolic systems in the body.

It controls the secretion of growth hormone (thymus) which affects the stature of the body, the thyroid which controls metabolism, the pancreas, Islets of Langerhans (**Paul Langerhans,** 1847-1888) which control the level of insulin and hence the amount of sugar in the bloodstream, the adrenal glands which release cortisone decreasing inflammation and adrenaline increasing heart rate, and the gonads in men and women affecting the level of testosterone and oestrogen.

At puberty, in the early to mid-teens there is a change in the amount of hormones secreted by the gonads leading to transformation of boys and girls into men and women with deepening of the voice and growth of facial hair in men and widening of the pelvis and enlargement of the breasts (mammary glands) in women. Secretion of milk occurs after the birth of a baby.

MSS: MUSCULO-SKELETAL SYSTEM

We form part of a group of animals known as vertebrates which have an endoskeleton or bones within the body, and there are features common to all.

There is a central vertebral column, from which arise the rib cage and four pentadactyl (five dactyls or digits) limbs. These are modified in different animals such that the upper arms become wings in birds and the toes turned around to be able to grip twigs and branches.

Humans have modified their great or 1st toes to align with the other metatarsals to enable us to run away from predators. Great apes still have the opposable toe to enable them to grip branches.

The bones meet at joints. There are fixed joints such as where the ribs meet the sternum or breastbone (cartilaginous joints), semi-fixed joints (fibrous joints) such as between the vertebrae or where the pelvic bones meet in the front, and mobile joints (synovial joints).

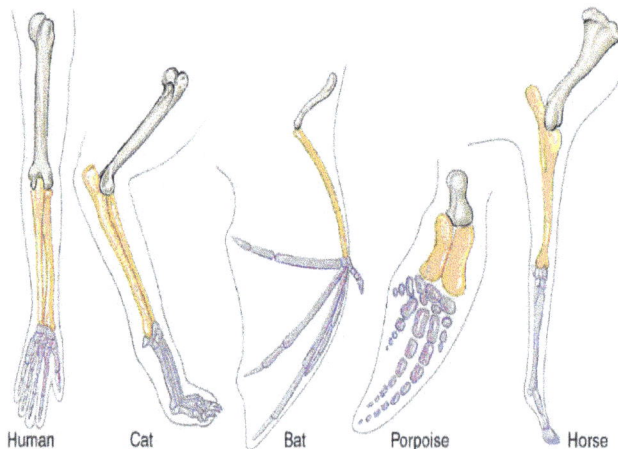

Human   Cat   Bat   Porpoise   Horse

The axial skeleton
The skull, vertebral column and rib cage. These bones protect the internal organs, as well as providing sites for muscle attachment.

Cervical vertebrae

Pectoral girdle
Clavicle
Scapula

Costal cartilages
These contribute to the elasticity of the thoracic wall

Radius
The head of this bone articulates with the humerus

Ulna

Carpus
The bones of the wrist articulate with the metacarpals, ulna and radius

Femur

The appendicular skeleton
Consists of the bones of the limbs, together with the pectoral and pelvic girdles which attach the limbs to the axial skeleton

Metatarsal bones

Skull
Protects the brain and the top of the spinal cord

Sternum
Cartilage is found where the ribs meet the sternum

Rib

Humerus
This is the largest bone in the upper limb and it articulates with the scapula at the shoulder joint

Hip bones

Sacrum

Pubic symphysis

Patella (knee cap)
Provides protection

Tibia (shin bone)

Fibula
Articulates with the tibia

Bone is actually living tissue – the skeleton has its own blood vessels and nerve supply. Up to 5 per cent of bone is recycled every week by its cells.

Spine of scapula
A thick ridge of bone which continues as the acromion of the shoulder

Infraspinous fossa of scapula

Lateral epicondyle of humerus
When the elbow joint is partially flexed, this can be felt

Iliac crest
A ridge that forms the rim of the fan-shaped ilium

Greater trochanter of femur
This protuberance occurs above the femur

Obturator foramen
A large aperture in the hip bone

Lateral malleolus of fibula
A projection at the lower end of the outer bone of the fibula

External occipital protuberance
This projection is usually easily palpable

Greater tubercle of humerus
A raised area at the lateral margin of the humerus

Spinous processes of vertebrae

Greater sciatic notch
A deep indentation of the ischium

Ischial tuberosity
A protuberance of the ischium

Lateral femoral condyle

Soleal line of tibia
A rough diagonal ridge of the shin bone

The bones of the human skeleton are rarely smooth. Markings are often found on bones where tendons, ligaments, and fasciae attach.

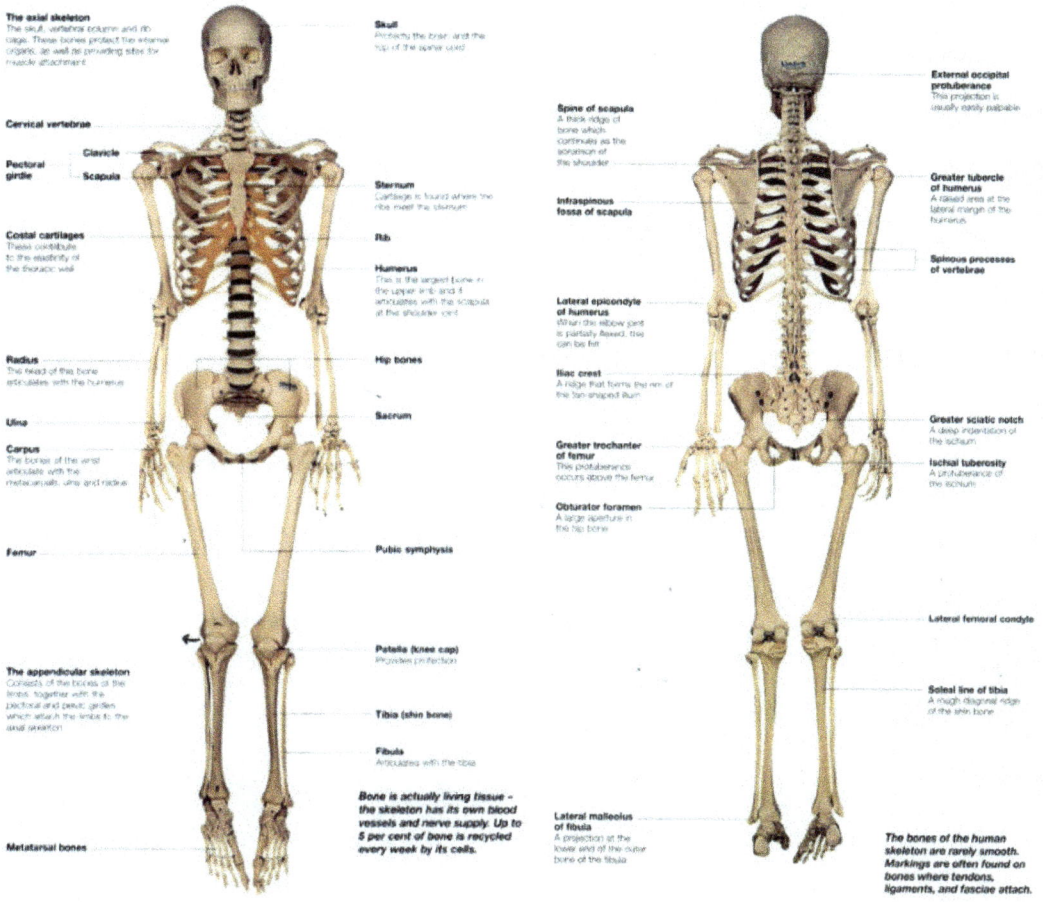

Above: in the human skeleton there are 33 vertebrae

In the human skeleton there are 33 vertebrae supporting a head at one end and articulating with the pelvis at the other with a rib cage, arms on either side, and legs.

A synovial joint is so-called because the bone ends are lined by hyaline cartilage which needs lubricating by the fluid secreted by the synovial membrane lining the capsule of the joint. The capsule is an enclosing membrane which is thickened in some parts by fibrous tissue called ligaments, restricting movements in some planes but not in others.

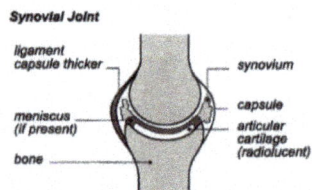

The cartilage is sometimes reinforced by a meniscus made of fibrocartilage (commonly called cartilages in the knee) which may be partial, as in the knee, or complete, as in the temporomandibular (jaw) joint. There are various types of joints such as ball and socket joints where free movement is allowed in various directions, hinge joints such as the elbow, combination joints such as the knee where some rotation is allowed, and facet joints in the spine.

There are pivot joints where the head meets the spinal column at the atlas (Cervical 1, or C1) to allow nodding, and swivel joints such as below the atlas (C1) with the dens of the axis vertebra (C2) to allow turning. The dens is formed from the ancient body of the atlas which has the two curved facets and the arch above. It is named after the Greek god who supported the world.

See in this picture below: Atlas is below, axis is above.

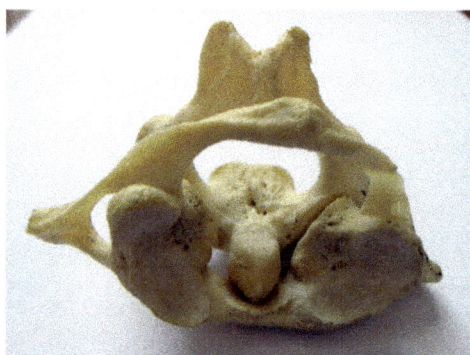

Notes:

There are some joints called saddle joints such as the base of the thumb which allow movement in different directions.

Bones are made of a fibrous tissue set in calcium hydroxyapatite (like chalk or coral). A decalcified bone is flexible such as this fibula:

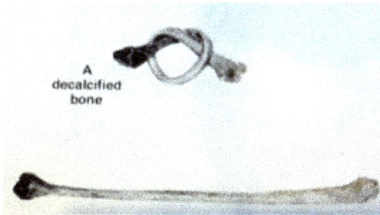

A decalcified bone

It is the calcium which blocks x-rays producing the shadow on the film first discovered by **Konrad Roentgen**, 1845-1923, in 1895. He called them x-rays as x is the mathematical symbol for unknown. He was experimenting with cathode ray tubes and had the wit to investigate a photographic plate fogged by unknown rays.

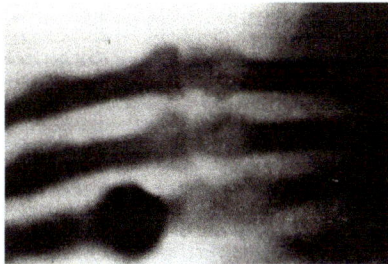

This is Roentgen's original x-ray of his wife's hand with her ring, taken after six minutes exposure. It created huge interest when he first published his results and over 1000 papers were produced in the year afterwards!

If barium salts were ingested, they were used to display the stomach and intestines.

Long bones are hollow to provide lightness with strength. Blood supply is via nutrient arteries and periosteum, a dense fibrous tissue which has the ability to make bone and is used to provide attachment to the muscles and tendons. The hollow is filled with marrow, which in children is haemopoietic producing red and white blood cells. In adults the marrow is replaced by liquid fat which in fractures may penetrate the vascular system producing a syndrome called fat embolism.

Notes:

There are two types of bony tissue.

Compact bone: this is dense bone made up of Haversian systems (see **Clopton Havers,** 1657-1702) with a lot of hydroxyapatite between the systems producing a dense appearance on x-rays.

Cancellous bone: this is made up of bony trabeculae usually aligned in the direction of force applied to the bone and consists of thin plates of bone interspersed with haemopoietic tissue.

Bone is similar to a Crunchie chocolate bar where the periosteum is the silver wrapping, the chocolate on the outside is the compact bone, and the honeycomb is the cancellous bone on the inside.

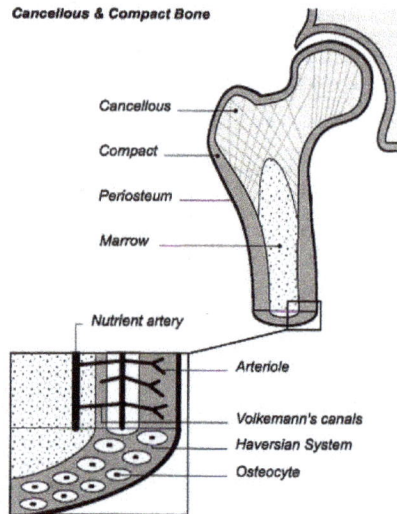

Cancellous & Compact Bone

Cancellous
Compact
Periosteum
Marrow
Nutrient artery
Arteriole
Volkemann's canals
Haversian System
Osteocyte

Bony growth occurs at the ends of long bones at the epiphysis which is made up of cartilage cells multiplying, hypertrophying, and calcifying, and being replaced by bone (metaphysis). The apophysis is the growth plate on the side of the bone, such as the front of the proximal tibia, or back of the calcaneus (heel bone). Remodelling occurs to ensure that the bone grows symmetrically.

This however is also determined by forces applied to the bone and because of the curled-up nature of the foetus in the uterus, the baby is born with bent legs which take about 12 months to straighten out.

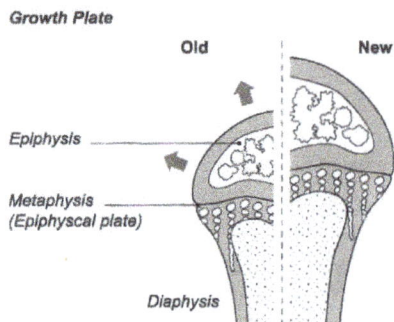

Growth Plate

Old   New

Epiphysis
Metaphysis (Epiphyscal plate)
Diaphysis

However, deficiencies of Vitamin D may also produce bowing of the legs called rickets. The diaphysis refers to the shaft of the bone.

Notes:

Bony growth ceases at the end of adolescence although the last epiphysis to close is the inner end of the clavicle around the age of 24.

Bone requires a blood supply and is in a constant state of removal and replacement according to the stresses laid upon it. Bone reacts to stress or irritation by either laying down bone due to over activity of the osteoblasts which are the cells that form bone and hardening of the bone is described as osteosclerosis (-sclerosis means hardening).

Bone is removed by the osteoclasts and this produces osteoporosis (generalised loss), or cysts (localised loss). Stable bone cells are called osteocytes. In some circumstances a mixed picture may appear in various disease processes such as Paget's disease where bone can be thickened and bent.

MUSCLES

There are various types of muscle fibres such as cardiac muscle which is specialised to provide rhythmic contraction continuously throughout life (see Image One).

There is smooth muscle which is found in the wall of the gut providing peristalsis and the movement of food through the alimentary canal. Smooth muscle is also found in some blood vessels which dilate when we blush and constrict; when we see a ghost for example (see Image Two).

The muscles that move the joints are called striated muscles because of their appearance under the microscope. They are formed into bundles that contract in unison in response to nervous stimuli. Energy is released in the cells and working muscles need a rich blood supply. If an accumulation of waste products occurs, cramp sets in.

They are extended by tendons of bundles of inelastic collagen fibres (similar to a rope) and form a strong attachment to bone.

Tendons slide within a sheath and are lubricated by synovial fluid. If a muscle contracts too violently, it can tear the muscle fibres themselves or the tendons (see Image Three).

Notes:

Microscopic structure of cardiac muscle

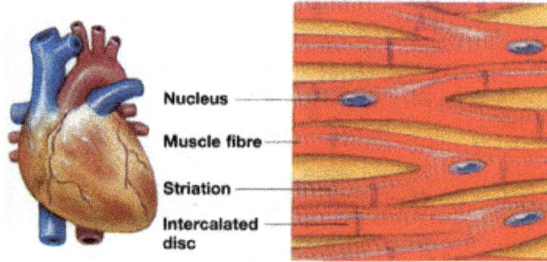

Nucleus

Muscle fibre

Striation

Intercalated disc

Above: Image One

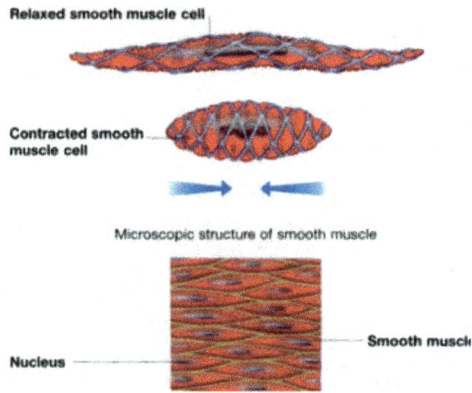

Relaxed smooth muscle cell

Contracted smooth muscle cell

Microscopic structure of smooth muscle

Nucleus

Smooth muscl[e]

Above: Image Two

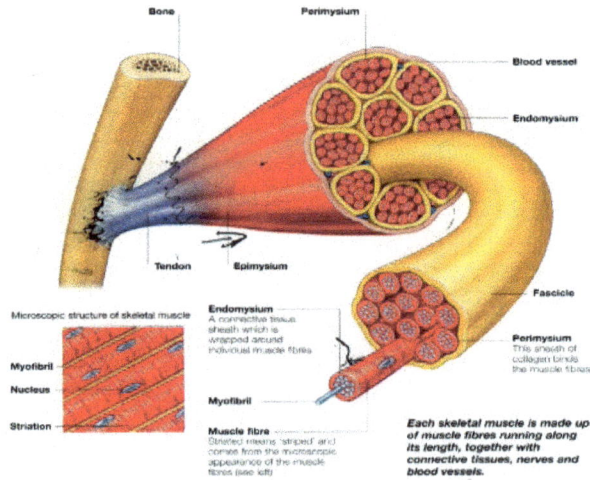

Bone

Perimysium

Blood vessel

Endomysium

Tendon

Epimysium

Fascicle

Microscopic structure of skeletal muscle

Myofibril

Nucleus

Striation

Endomysium
A connective tissue sheath which is wrapped around individual muscle fibres

Myofibril

Muscle fibre
Striated means 'striped' and comes from the microscopic appearance of the muscle fibres (see left)

Perimysium
This sheath of collagen binds the muscle fibres

Each skeletal muscle is made up of muscle fibres running along its length, together with connective tissues, nerves and blood vessels.

Above: Image Three

The image below on the left is a woodcut of **Andreas Versalius,** 1514–1564, who made a major contribution to anatomy when he published his book *De Humani Corporis Fabricia* in 1543. The image on the right is taken from that book.

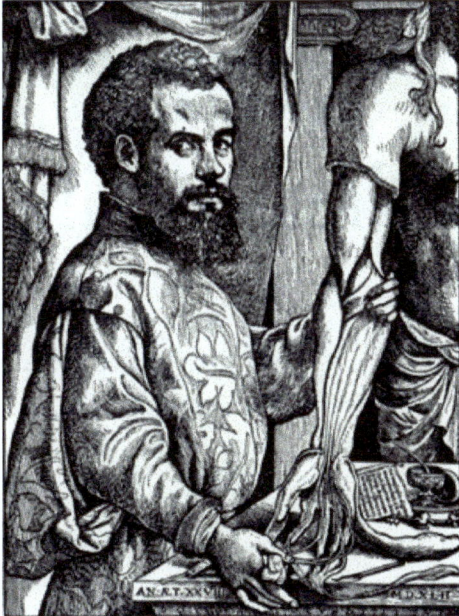

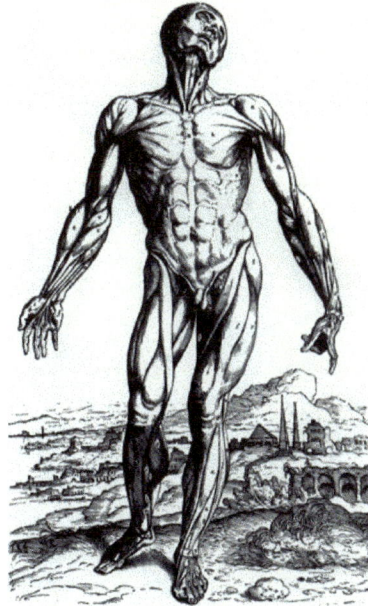

WHAT CAN GO WRONG

This is called **PATHOLOGY**.

It applies to all the different systems and affects their functions. Sometimes the developing cells do not grow correctly, and these conditions are **CONGENITAL**. Often, it is based on faulty genes and more and more conditions are now being diagnosed and sometimes corrected in utero.

Because the zygote divides into two after fertilisation then again and again, it means the embryo is formed in two halves which can be seen in the shallow cleft in the upper lip (philtrum) once the baby is born. Sometimes, this persists as a <u>cleft palate and/or lip</u>.

<u>Spina bifida</u> which may allow the spinal cord and dura to protrude from the body, known as a meningo-myelocoele, may render the baby paraplegic (loss of function in the lower limbs). It may also be associated with hydrocephalus where there is a blockage in the ventricular system in the brain causing swelling of the head.

<u>Down's Syndrome</u>, see **John Down,** 1828-1896, or Mongolism where the child is mentally deficient.

<u>Developmental dysplasia of the hip</u> is where the head of the femur does not fit the socket.

<u>Talipes equino-varus</u> or club foot.

<u>Achondroplasia</u> or dwarfism.

<u>Osteogenesis imperfecta</u> or brittle bones; the bones are more fragile.

<u>Cerebral palsy</u>, then early spasticity, or writhing (athetosis) movements, although this may be associated with another cause such as brain damage from lack of oxygen or trauma.

ACQUIRED conditions come on throughout life. Many words in medicine have prefixes or suffixes to clarify their meaning and most are based on Latin or Greek. They affect the different systems in the body. The four most common causes are **inflammation, trauma, neoplasia, and degeneration**.

INFLAMMATION, INFLAMMATORY (-ITIS):

Can be acute or chronic. Tissues react to irritation such as from bacteria, (infection), or chemicals by the production of fluid and the invasion of white cells (macrophages). Pus is made up of this fluid, and dead bacteria. A collection of pus is called an abscess. It may come on suddenly or persist.

Notes:

The suffix -itis is applied to the organ affected, such as tonsillitis, appendicitis, osteomyelitis. 2000 years ago, the Greek, **Aulus Celsus, 53BCE-7CE,** described the following as the effects of inflammation:

- Rubor, redness
- Dolor, pain
- Calor, heat
- Tumor, swelling, to which may be added
- Loss of function

One of my heroes in medicine is **Ambroise Paré,** 1510-1590. When he was a young doctor, he joined the army as a surgeon. There were various wars being fought in Europe at that time.

It is better to let him describe in his own words what happened:

I had not yet seen gunshot wounds at the first dressing. I had read in Jean De Vigo's book "Of Wounds in General" Chapter 8, that wounds made by firearms partake of venomosity, by reason of the gunpowder, and for their cure he bids you cauterise them with oil of elder, scalding hot, mixed with a little treacle.

And to make no mistake, before I would use this said oil, knowing it was to bring great pain to the patient I asked first, before I applied it, what the other surgeons used for the first dressing; which was to put the said oil, boiling well, into the wounds, and tents and setons [drains]; wherefore I took courage to do as they did.

At last, my oil ran short; and I was compelled instead of it, to apply a digestive made of yolk of eggs, oil of roses and turpentine.

In the night I could not sleep in quiet, fearing some default in not cauterising, lest I should find those, to whom I have not applied the said oil, dead from the poison of their wounds; which made me rise very early to visit them; where, beyond my expectation, I found that they to whom I had applied my digestive had suffered but little pain in their wounds without inflammation or swelling, having rested fairly well that night.

The others to whom the boiling oil was applied, I found feverish, with great pain, and swelling around the edges of their wounds. Then I resolved never more to cruelly burn these poor men with gunshot wounds.

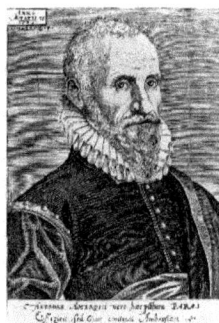

This is a very good description of the inflammatory reaction to boiling oil, and also a lesson to not believe everything that one reads in established textbooks or is taught.

TRAUMA, TRAUMATIC:

This is injury to a tissue with the result depending on the force and the tissues to which it is applied. For example:

Soft tissue may be bruised, or bone broken, often referred to as a fracture. Signs of inflammation are present.

Bleeding into the tissues produces a haematoma (swelling) and colour changes as the blood is broken down over a period of two to three weeks.

Joints may be sprained or dislocated, where the ligaments and capsule are stretched and torn.

The wound may be closed or open and the latter is more liable to infection, as the skin is torn.

Major injuries involve several systems and are life threatening. Urgent treatment will be considered in the next chapter.

NEOPLASIA, NEOPLASTIC:

Neo [new] and *Plasia* [growth]

New growth of tissues independent of normal control (tumour — which really means swelling). The body does not recognise that they may be harmful and feeds them; often causing death in malignant tumours that are not successfully treated.

MALIGNANT (-carcinoma, -sarcoma):

These tumours invade the surrounding tissue and metastasise or spread to distant parts via lymphatics or the blood stream. These secondary deposits are known as metastases or secondaries.

They can be graded from 1-4 or early and late (where spread has occurred).

Carcinoma: This usually applied to the tissues derived from the ectoderm and endoderm such as squamous cell carcinoma of the skin, adenocarcinoma of the breast, or of the stomach. Early spread is to the lymph nodes and later via the blood stream.

Notes:

Sarcoma: This usually applies to tissues derived from the mesoderm such as fibrosarcoma, osteosarcoma or myosarcoma. Early spread is via the blood stream. The effects depend on the rate of growth of the tumour and how quickly it spreads.

Superficial tumours are more quickly diagnosed, and treatment is often effective before they have spread.

Cancer is a word commonly, but wrongly, used and creates fear, as not all malignant tumours are fatal.

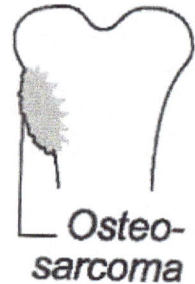

Osteo-sarcoma

BENIGN (-oma):

This is a tumour which remains localised to the area. The suffix -oma is applied to the tissue such as lipoma (a fatty tumour), fibroma (a fibrous tumour). The effects produced depend on the situation. Swelling may be visible, and pain may be produced from pressure on sensitive surrounding tissue. These often do not need a biopsy, unless the diagnosis is in doubt.

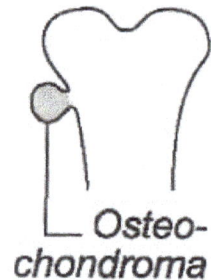

Osteo-chondroma

DEGENERATION (-osis):

This is ageing of the tissues and occurs to us all. Spondylosis means degeneration of the spine, and arthrosis degeneration of a joint (arthrus); although arthritis is the more commonly-used term.

This spine is from the British Museum's Mummy section and shows a 2000-year-old spine with marked degenerative changes, with narrowing of the disc spaces and lipping, spurs, or osteophytes. I am sure he would have had back ache!!

Sclerosis means hardening and is seen where the bone has to take an increased load such as in softening of the discs in the spine as shown.

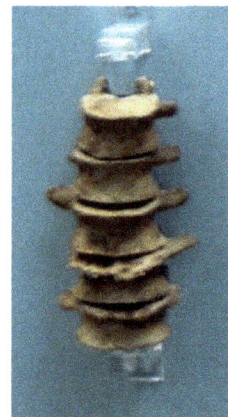

Arteriosclerosis is the hardening of the arteries by deposits of calcium in the walls lining them, and narrowing by deposits of fats, such as cholesterol, called plaques. This can start in your early twenties, which was found in autopsies of soldiers killed by wounds back in the Korean war in the 1950s.

Notes:

This can lead to heart attacks, (myocardial infarcts, or MI, in doctor speak) and strokes (cerebro-vascular accidents, or CVA). Stenosis means narrowing, such as associated with the narrowing of the exit foramina seen in chronic degeneration in the spine.

Osteoarthritis (OA) is the common term for joint disease. Degeneration commences in the articular cartilage; see page 24. It is common in the weight bearing joints, such as the hip and knee, and in the joints of the spine.

METABOLIC:

This involves the energy and chemical processes in the body such as too much uric acid from the breakdown of amino acids producing gout and crystals in the joint causing pain. A healthy diet is needed to prevent deficiency diseases such as scurvy from a lack of vitamin C (found in oranges, lemons, and limes) rickets (bowlegs) from a lack of vitamin D). Sailors in the British Navy in the 18th century were known as limeys from the use of rum and sugar to hide the sourness of the limes.

ENDOCRINE:

This affects the various glands in the body such as an overactive pituitary producing excess growth in children with gigantism, or, in adults, acromegaly. Diabetes is altered pancreatic production of insulin moderating blood sugar levels.

IMMUNOLOGICAL:

Disorders of the immune system such as rheumatoid arthritis or AIDS (auto-immune deficiency syndrome).

PYSCHOSOMATIC:

This is where the person believes there is a problem, when there is no organic cause and when carried to excess is commonly called Munchausen's syndrome. Mental illness is due to disorders of the psychological system.

IATROGENIC:

This is a medical complication, such as injecting a nerve producing damage.

IDIOPATHIC:

This is where no cause is found.

HOW TO
TREAT IT

This depends on establishing a **DIAGNOSIS,** or cause of a condition. A diagnosis is based on history, examination, and investigation (symptoms, signs, tests). Various conditions are considered, and a list of priorities drawn up (differential diagnosis). Common things occur commonly.

SYMPTOMS:

These are complaints made by the patient and the commonest in musculo-skeletal conditions is pain. Different people are affected differently, and some people are more stoic than others. Pain is an emotive term and can be superficial or deep. Superficial pain often produces words like burning or scalding, a feeling like ants under the skin or sharp like a pinprick. Deep pain uses words like aching or crushing. Litigation has been shown to prolong symptoms in some cases, possibly due to an unconscious desire to punish the other party. However, they do not always resolve when the case is settled.

Sometimes patients fall into the sick role syndrome where they get attention from other members of the family that they may not have had before.

Sometimes symptoms are fabricated as in the Munchausen syndrome and doctors are led on various wild goose chases that may even involve surgery, before it is recognised.

In writing up a case history it is usually under different headings such as:

- PC: Present complaints
- HPI: History of the present illness
- FH: Family history
- SH: Social history

SIGNS:

These are findings on examination.

GENERAL EXAMINATION:

A doctor usually starts an observation as soon as a patient enters the consulting room, and much can be learned from the demeanour, facial expression, and behaviour.

A person can be seen to be in agony by the expression on their face.

Notes:

Chronic pain can cause deep shadows under the eyes and a gaunt expression. When faced with such a person who says there is little wrong with them, a doctor must beware.

Similarly, a person who describes chronic pain but is not obviously in pain and who has a normal appearance with little to show on their face may be just seeking attention.

Much can be learnt by how the patient describes their condition and their tone of voice.

LOCAL EXAMINATION:
Look — inspection — the part may be red and swollen suggesting an infection.

Feel — palpation — gentle pressure may cause acute pain or there may be rebound pain when the hand is lifted suddenly from the abdomen, for example, in appendicitis.

Move — percussion — tapping an area may produce a dull sound; or moving a joint may cause pain.

Hear — auscultation — sometimes joints creak when moved or there may be crackles and wheezes heard when listening to the lungs. [The stethoscope was invented to protect the modesty of female patients when examining the chest.]

The following terms are used to help to understand the location of the problem:

- Anterior (ventral) is in front, posterior (dorsal) behind, and lateral to the side.
- All joints are at 0° in the erect position except during pronation and supination where, with the elbow flexed at 90° and thumb up, is 0°.

Notes:

Positions   Movements

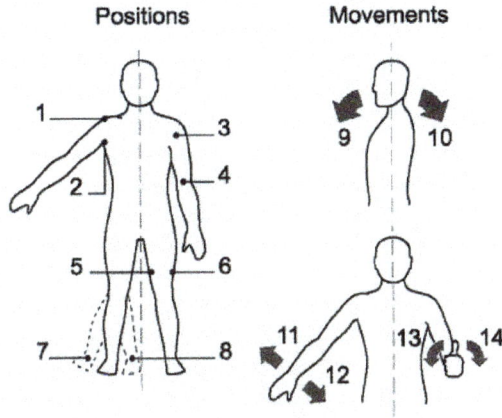

1.	**Supra-/superior**	Above
2.	**Infra-/inferior**	Below
3.	**Proximal**	Towards the top
4.	**Distal**	Towards the bottom
5.	**Medial**	On the inner side
6.	**Lateral**	On the outer side
7.	**Valgus**	Away from the midline
8.	**Varus**	Towards the midline
9.	**Flexion**	Bending forwards
10.	**Extension**	Bending backwards
11.	**Abduction**	Movement away from the midline
12.	**Adduction**	Movement towards the midline
13.	**Pronation**	Rotating inwards
14.	**Supination**	Rotating outwards

Notes:

TESTS:

If the diagnosis is in doubt, or to confirm the diagnosis, tests are carried out either on an outpatient or inpatient basis. They are expensive and should not be ordered indiscriminately.

X-ray: AP (antero-posterior or front to back), lateral (sideways), and oblique views are necessary to obtain the best information, e.g, cervical spine.

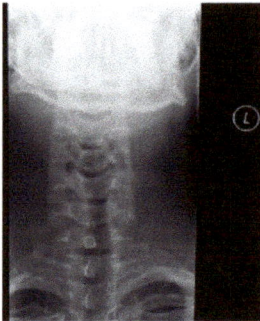

AP

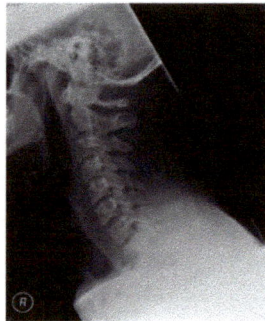

Lateral

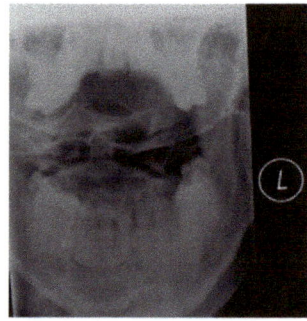

Open mouth
(peg view as the jaw obscures the uppermost vertebrae)

Blood: A full blood screen to include red cell count, white cell count, ESR (erythrocyte sedimentation rate: the rate at which red cells drop in plasma), blood chemistry e.g., raised uric acid in gout. Blood culture if infection is suspected.

Urine: Blood, protein, organisms, and crystals.

Sputum: Culture, cytology.

Notes:

SPECIAL INVESTIGATIONS:

Computerised Axial Tomography (CAT) also (CT): A special x-ray showing sections through the body.

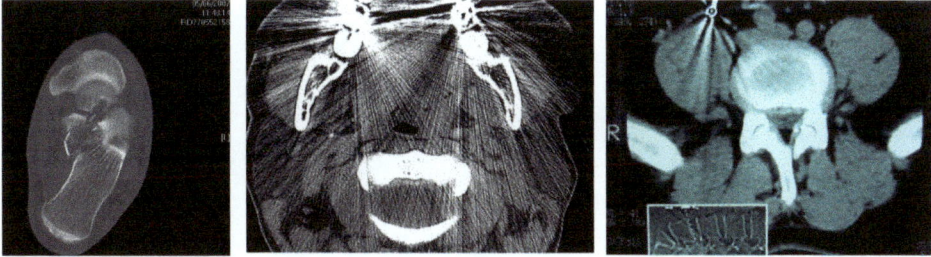

This shows a fracture on the inner side of the calcaneus or heel bone.

Here is a CT of the upper cervical spine showing scatter due to metallic fillings in the teeth.

This is an unusual scatter from a small linear object just visible in front of the vertebrae on the bottom of the picture and is hollow. It was the appendix with barium from a barium enema some days before.

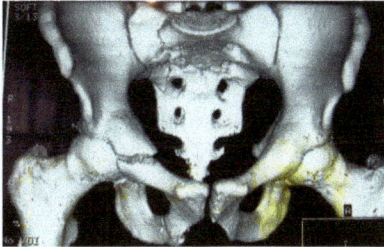

Above: 3D imaging is now available. Note the fracture below in the right pelvis (acetabulum).

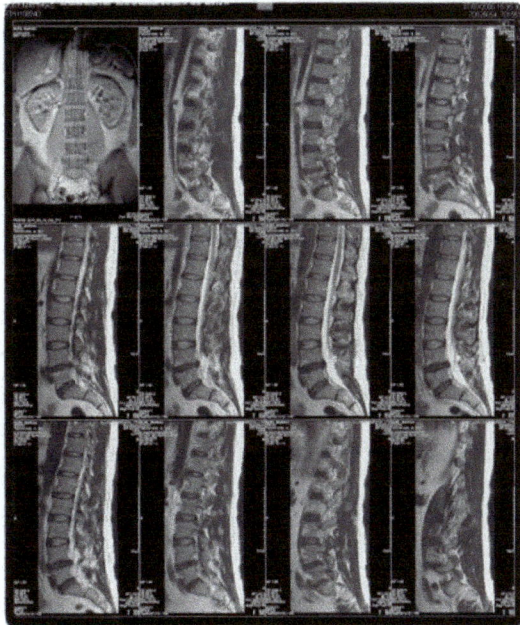

Above: Magnetic Resonance Imaging (MRI). Resonance of water molecules in the magnetic field shows soft tissues in vertical and horizontal planes. 3D images are now available. This shows a series of cuts in the sagittal plane of the lumber spine from one side to the other. Note the disc bulge at L4/5

Radio Isotope Scanning: Uptake by bone of isotopes showing hot or cold areas of increased or decreased bone activity. It is filtered and excreted by the kidneys within a few hours.

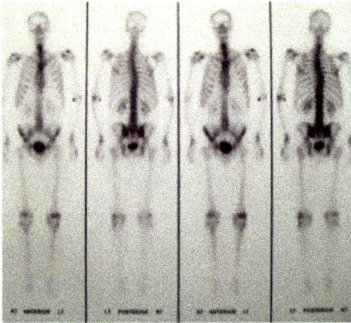

The image above is normal apart from showing a slight scoliosis or twist of the spine. Note the bladder in the pelvis.

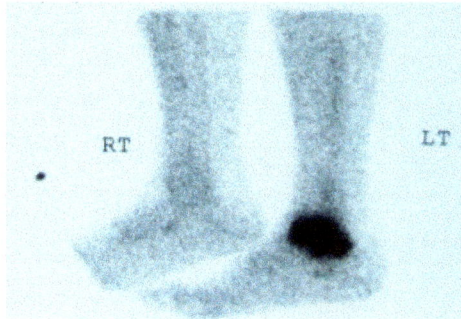

The image above shows the author's "hot" ankle with inflammation from gouty arthritis.

Contrast medium X-ray: Injection of radio opaque material into a joint shows soft tissue.

Arthroscopy: Looking into a joint.

Arteriography: Injection of radio opaque material into an artery measuring blood flow through an area. Note the pinching of the upper and lower arteries in this arteriogram of a heart. Stents were inserted (see image to the right).

Bone mineral density: Tests where the bones have lost or added calcium.

Electromyography (EMG) or Nerve Conduction Study (NCS): Tests conductivity of nerves.

Ultrasound (US): High frequency sound waves show soft tissues. Note the face of this baby in the US of a pregnant woman near term (see image to the right).

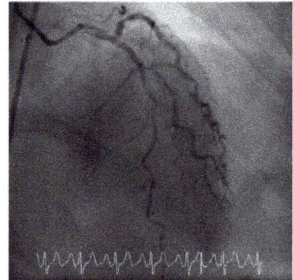

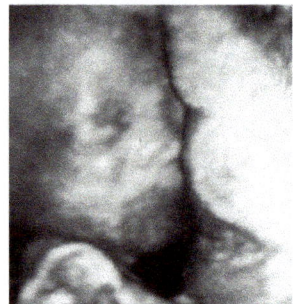

Notes:

Having made a diagnosis **TREATMENT** is considered.

The two words that summarise treatment are kind and nous (pronounced nowse). To be kind to someone means being gentle and treating them with courtesy and compassion. Nous means using one's common sense and initiative.

Before treatment is commenced the **PROGNOSIS** or outcome of the condition must be considered, as nature has a strong inbuilt mechanism towards healing, and practitioners must assist nature as much as possible.

Results and complications (side effects) of treatment must be known. The cure should not be worse than the disease! Prevention is better than cure, e.g., anti-coagulants to prevent Deep Vein Thrombosis (DVT) and Pulmonary Embolism (PE) following major surgery, antibiotics against infections, or vaccinations against tetanus for example.

General:

The patient must be treated as a whole person and includes not only the management of the acute situation but also convalescence and final recovery. This applies to mental health as well.

Local:

Conservative (or non-operative):

This depends on which system is involved with what pathology. "Rest, Diet, and Drugs", for example, involves the use of anti-biotics for infection, analgesics (pain relief), anti-inflammatories (often called NSAIDS — Non-Steroidal Anti-Inflammatory Drugs) for degenerative or inflammatory conditions such as rheumatoid arthritis, insulin for diabetics, massage, manipulation, and so on, and may be carried out by various disciplines.

Many fractures can be managed this way especially in children as growth will often correct some deformity (but not rotation). When treating someone with a broken arm for example, one must treat the patient and not the x-ray. The principles are:

- **Reduce:** Restore the alignment and angulation as soon as possible if a joint is dislocated.
- **Hold:** Splints or plaster (which may be plastic), or internal fixation with screws and plates.
- **Use:** Restore and maintain function.

Notes:

Operative:

In the case of surgery, pre- and post-operative care are as important as the operation itself.

Various suffixes are used to denote operations:

- ostomy/-otomy	(cutting into) such as tracheostomy (making a hole in the trachea), osteotomy (cutting into a bone)
- lysis	(freeing of) such as tenolysis (freeing of a tendon), neurolysis (freeing of a nerve)
- plasty	(refashioning) such as arthroplasty (making a new joint), mammoplasty (refashioning a breast)
- ectomy	(removal of) such as gastrectomy (removal of the stomach)
- scopy	(looking into) such as arthroscopy (looking into a joint-arthrus), laparoscopy (looking into the abdomen)
- desis	(fusion) such as arthrodesis (where two bones are fused together, and the joint becomes immobile)

Treatment involves a team which includes doctors, nurses, physiotherapists, occupational therapists, social workers, osteopaths, chiropractors, and paramedical personnel, and can take place either at home or in hospital.

A hospital is like a small city and efficient running requires the help of cooks, porters, engineers, telephonists, secretarial staff, cleaners, gardeners, and not least of all administrators and, nowadays, security personnel. There is pressure to minimise costs, but this must not be allowed to minimise the quality of treatment although costs must be borne in mind. Treatment does entail side effects, and treatment must not be worse than the disease. Nature, by and large, helps healing.

Before leaving treatment, the placebo effect must be considered. This is where treatment with no chemical or surgical benefit is prescribed, and often helps in about 30% of cases, even when the patients know that a placebo is being used. It is a case of mind over matter.

Notes:

THE MANAGEMENT OF MAJOR ACCIDENTS

1. **The management at scene and transport to hospital:** This is usually left to the paramedics who arrive, but prior to their arrival it is important to establish an airway to maintain respiration and to arrest bleeding. The spinal cord should be protected by keeping the patient still until a hard collar can be applied and a spinal board fitted.

2. **Treatment in Accident and Emergency:** The ATLS (Advanced Trauma and Life Support) system is followed (or EMST — Early Management of Severe Trauma — in Australasia).

PRIMARY SURVEY:

A	**Airway** (cervical spine control)
B	**Breathing** and ventilation
C	**Circulation**. Control haemorrhage. Blood pressure. Pulse. An iv (intra-venous) cannula is inserted, and fluids commenced to prevent shock
D	**Disability** (neurological status) A　　Alert V　　Responds to vocal stimuli P　　Responds to painful stimuli U　　Unconscious
E	**Exposure** (undress patient, keep warm)
R	**Resuscitate**

Notes:

SECONDARY SURVEY:

1. History
2. Examination: Glasgow Coma Scale (GCS)
   - Normal (15)
   - Eye opening (4)
   - Verbal response (5)
   - Motor response (6)
3. Treatment: repair damage – priorities
   - Ruptured spleen takes precedence over fractured femur. It may involve several disciplines.

CARE OF THE DYING PATIENT

1. **Analgesia:** do not withhold opiates
2. **Good nursing:** soft pillows and sheets, TLC (tender loving care)
3. **Do not resuscitate:** death is a release

In this regard there is another story from Paré's war journal:

We entered pell mell into the city and in a stable where we thought to lodge our horses, we found four dead soldiers and three propped against the wall. They neither saw, heard nor spoke and their clothes were still smouldering, burned with gunpowder. As I was looking on them with pity, there came an old soldier who asked me if there were any way to cure them: I said, No. Then he went up to them and cut their throats gently and without ill will. I told him he was a villain: he answered he prayed God when he was in such a plight, he might find someone to do the same for him, that he should not linger in misery.

Later, when Paré was much older, he was sent by the King of France to look after Monsieur Le Marquis d'Aurel, a young man who was dying because of a compound fracture of his thigh following a fall from a horse. Paré wrote in his journal:

I found him in high fever, his eyes deep sunken, with a moribund and yellowish face, his tongue dry and parched, and the whole body wasted and lean, the voice low, as of a man very near death.

I found his thigh much inflamed, suppurating, and ulcerated, discharging a greenish and very offensive sanies. I probed it with a silver probe, wherewith

Notes:

I found a large cavity in the middle of the thigh and others around the knee, also several scales of bone, some loose, others not. There was a large bedsore; he could rest neither day nor night; and had no appetite to eat, but very thirsty.

Seeing and considering all these great complications and the vital powers thus broken down, truly, I was very sorry I had come to see him because it seemed to me there was very little hope, he could escape death.

All the same, to give him courage and good hope, I told him I would soon set him on his legs by the grace of God and the help of his physicians and surgeons.

Having seen him, I went for a walk in the garden, and prayed God to show me this grace, that he should recover, and to bless our hands and our mendicants to cure such a complication of disease. I turned in my mind what measures I must take to this end.

They called me to dinner. I came into the kitchen, and there I saw, taken out of a great pot, half a sheep, a quarter of veal, three great pieces of beef, two fowls, and a very large piece of bacon with abundance of good herbs.

Then I said to myself that the broth of the pot would be full of juices and very nourishing.

After dinner, we began our conversation, all physicians, and surgeons together, in the presence of Monsieur le Duc d'Ascot, and some other gentlemen who were with him.

I began to say to the surgeons that I was astonished that they had not made incisions in the patient's thigh, seeing as it was suppurating, and the thick matter in it very foetid and offensive, showing it had long been pent up there; and I had found with the probe caries of the bone and scales of bone already loose.

They answered me, never would he consent to it; and indeed, that it was near two months, since they had been able to get clean sheets on the bed, and that one scarce dared to touch the coverlet, so great was his pain.

Then I said, to cure him, we must touch something else than the coverlet of his bed. Each said what he thought of the malady of the patient, and in conclusion they all held it hopeless.

I told them that there was still some hope, because he was young, and God and Nature sometime do what seem to physicians and surgeons impossible.

I proposed three incisions for drainage, fomentations, a clean bed, hot water bottles, a pillow so adjusted as to relieve pressure on the bedsore, dusting powders, an opiate to ensure good sleep at night and a moderate allowance of wine.

To help sleep artificial rain must be made by pouring water from a height into a cauldron so that it made the soothing sound of falling rain.

The diet should include raw eggs, plums stewed in wine and sugar, good broth from the pot, fowls and other roast meats easy to digest, good bread that was neither too stale or too new.

Medicines prescribed must be properly flavoured, to disguise their taste.

This, my discourse was well approved by the physicians and surgeons. The consultation ended, and we went back to the patient, and I made three openings in his thigh. Two or three hours later, I got a bed made near his old one, with clean white sheets on it; then a strong man put him into it and he was thankful to be taken out of his foul stinking bed.

Soon afterwards, he asked to sleep; which he did for nearly four hours; and everybody in the house began to feel happy, and especially his brother...

Then, when I saw him beginning to get well, I told him that he was to have viols and violins, and a buffoon to make him laugh, which he did.

In a month, we got him into a chair; and he had himself carried about his garden, and to the door of his Chateau to watch people passing.

The villagers for two or three leagues round, now that they could see him, came on holidays to sing, and dance, a regular crowd of light-hearted country folk, rejoicing in his convalescence, all glad to see him not without plenty of laughter and plenty of drink. He always gave them a hogshead of beer; and they all drank his health with a will.

In six weeks, he began to stand a little on crutches, and to put on flesh and to get a good natural colour. He wanted to go to Beaumont, his brother's place; and was taken thither in a carrying chair; by eight men at a time.

And the peasants, in the villages through which we passed, when they knew it was Monsieur le Marquis, fought who should carry him and insisted that he should drink with them; and it was only beer, but they would have given Hippocras, if there had been any; and all were glad to see him and prayed God for him.

Paré said: Je le traité, Dieu le Guérit ... I treated him, God cured him.

Notes:

This algorithm is a summary:

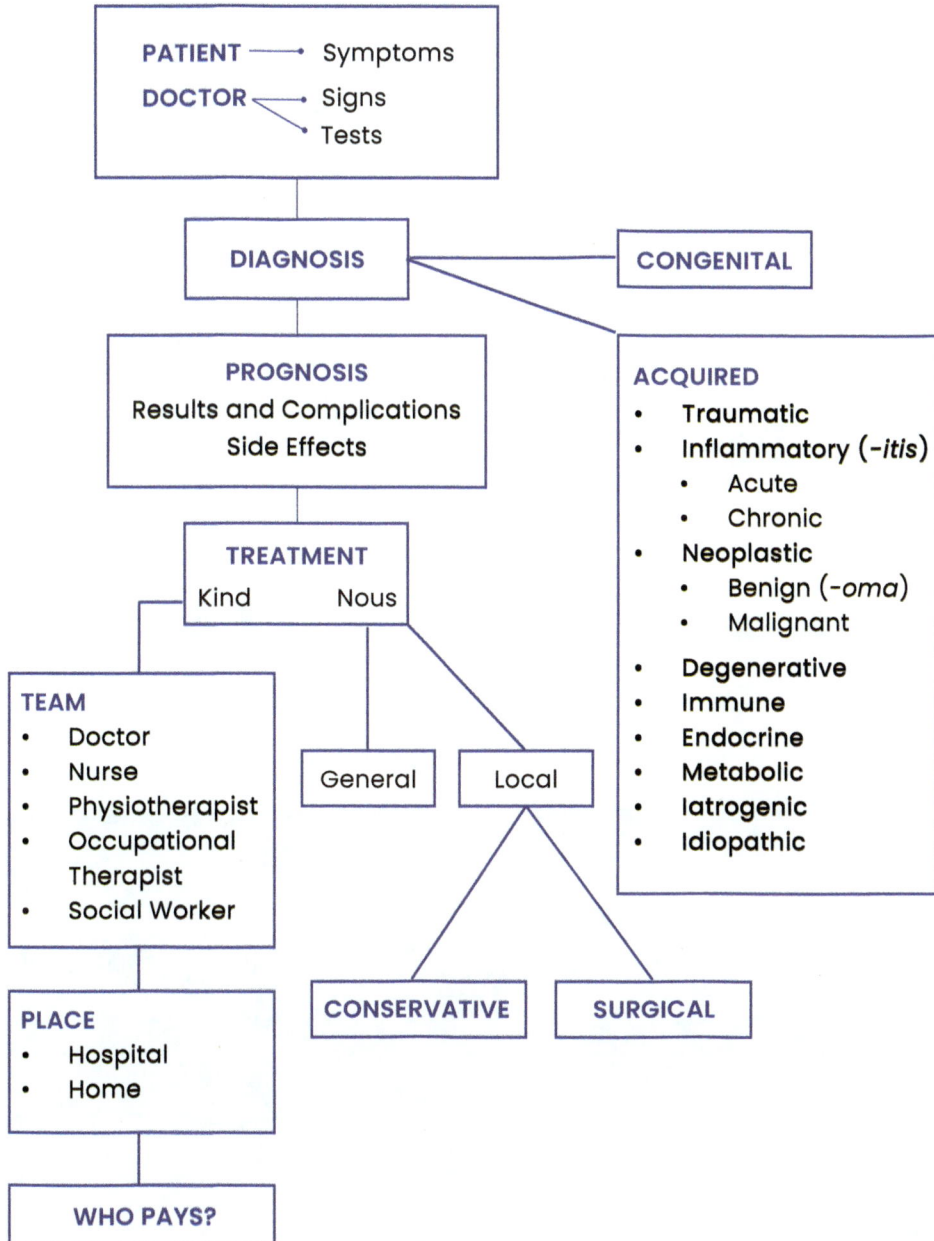

```
┌─────────────────────────────────┐
│  PATIENT ──────▸ Symptoms       │
│                                 │
│  DOCTOR ◂──────  Signs          │
│           ╲────▸ Tests          │
└─────────────────────────────────┘
                │
        ┌───────────────┐                    ┌──────────────┐
        │  DIAGNOSIS    │────────────────────│ CONGENITAL   │
        └───────────────┘                    └──────────────┘
                │
        ┌───────────────────────────┐        ┌──────────────────────────────┐
        │      PROGNOSIS            │        │ ACQUIRED                     │
        │ Results and Complications │        │  •  Traumatic                │
        │      Side Effects         │        │  •  Inflammatory (-itis)     │
        └───────────────────────────┘        │       •  Acute               │
                │                             │       •  Chronic             │
        ┌───────────────┐                     │  •  Neoplastic               │
        │  TREATMENT    │                     │       •  Benign (-oma)       │
        │ Kind    Nous  │                     │       •  Malignant           │
        └───────────────┘                     │  •  Degenerative             │
         │          │                         │  •  Immune                   │
┌──────────────────┐│                         │  •  Endocrine                │
│ TEAM             ││  ┌─────────┐ ┌───────┐  │  •  Metabolic                │
│  •  Doctor       ││  │ General │ │ Local │  │  •  Iatrogenic               │
│  •  Nurse        ││  └─────────┘ └───────┘  │  •  Idiopathic               │
│  •  Physiotherapist                         └──────────────────────────────┘
│  •  Occupational │
│     Therapist    │
│  •  Social Worker│
└──────────────────┘
         │
┌──────────────────┐    ┌──────────────────┐ ┌──────────────┐
│ PLACE            │    │  CONSERVATIVE    │ │  SURGICAL    │
│  •  Hospital     │    └──────────────────┘ └──────────────┘
│  •  Home         │
└──────────────────┘
         │
┌──────────────────┐
│   WHO PAYS?      │
└──────────────────┘
```

PART ONE:

Congenital Anomalies and Growth Disorders

DEVELOPMENTAL DYSPLASIA OF THE HIP (DDH)

This used to be called Congenital Dislocation of the Hip (CDH). The more accepted term is a developmental alteration in the growth of the ball and socket joint. Again, there is the use of Latin *dys* meaning faulty and *plasia* meaning growth.

This occurs in about 1/1000 live births and is more commonly seen in females than males in the ratio of 3:1.

CAUSE

It is thought to be due to laxity of the capsule of the hip possibly due to the transfer of hormones across the placental barrier. This causes generalised ligamentous laxity, and most babies are able to bring their foot up to their mouth to suck their big toe as easily as they can suck their thumb. They all have flat feet when they first stand up and gradually the arch develops as they grow, and the ligaments become stronger.

Most babies have clicking hips at birth but only 1/1000 proceed to a clinical condition. If the hip remains out of socket, then changes occur in both the socket and the head of the femur, producing a shallow socket or acetabulum and a small head of femur.

DIAGNOSIS IN NEONATE

Ortolani Test: The hips are abducted with the knees bent and a click or clunk can be felt and heard as the hip goes in and out of socket. Sometimes there is an alteration in the skin creases in the buttock, but this is an inconclusive sign as extra creases are not uncommon.

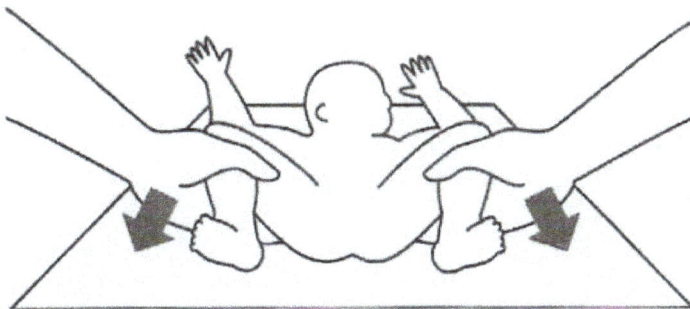

Notes:

If the condition is suspected an ultrasound scan will commonly show whether the hip is in or is not out of socket.

Because the bones do not show on an x-ray until three months of age, x-rays are not helpful before then. They are rarely performed these days.

In this diagram, note the angle the neck makes with the long axis of the femur (normal 130°).

This becomes more obtuse as the hip grows in a dislocated hip and is called a coxa valga.

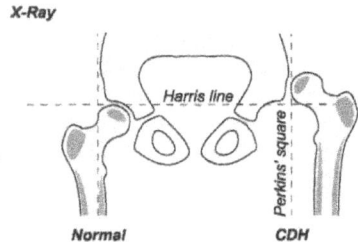

X-Ray

Harris line

Perkins' square

Normal   CDH

TREATMENT

Early:

Provided the hip is reduced and held within the socket then normal growth will usually resolve the problem. The early treatment is to maintain the hip with the knees out from the side or in abduction using double nappies or various forms of harness (Pavlik) or **Dennis Browne**, 1892-1967, splints. Sometimes the baby needs to be admitted to hospital for traction with gradual abduction of the hip such that the legs are widely out from the side and when ultrasound or x-rays show the hip is reduced, a plaster cast is applied.

Late:

If the diagnosis is missed at birth and is not made until the child is walking, then surgical treatment is often necessary. Often the child will walk with a waddling gait, or a limp if only one hip is involved. Because the tendons holding the hip in towards the side are tight, these are cut in what is called an adductor tenotomy.

Sometimes the hip is opened and the cartilaginous rim around the hip called the limbus is everted to go over the outside of the head of the femur rather than preventing its reduction.

Sometimes it is necessary to alter the shape of the socket through performing an osteotomy or cutting into the pelvis (described by **Robert Salter**, 1924-2010, of Toronto) and sometimes it is necessary to alter the angle of the neck and shaft of the femur by doing a femoral osteotomy.

Notes:

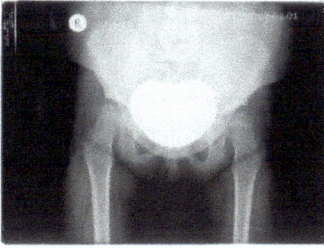

Note here (top left) the coxa valga on each side. This child was six years old with a late diagnosis at two years of age, but then appropriately treated.

Sometimes a dysplastic hip is not diagnosed until the 20s or 30s due to aching in the hip or referred pain to the knee and is picked up on x-ray where there is a loss of the neck shaft angle.

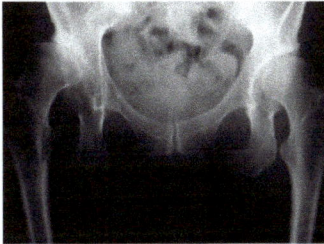

The head of the femur (bottom left) is supported by a neck and the angle between the shaft of the femur and the neck is usually 130°. A more open angle alters the forces acting on the hip producing arthritic changes through the surface of the femur and the adjacent acetabulum.

Treatment may be either by femoral osteotomy or more commonly by hip replacement if degenerative change is advanced and the symptoms are severe.

This (top right) was a hip replacement in a 37-year-old woman using a metal-on-metal replacement known as the Birmingham hip. 10 years later she had to have it revised to a more conventional prosthesis.

Note the left hip is slowly showing some changes of arthritis with sclerosis in the acetabulum (bottom right).

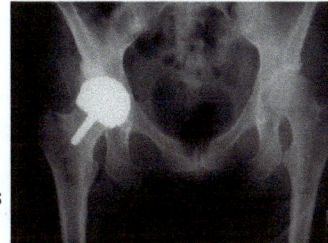

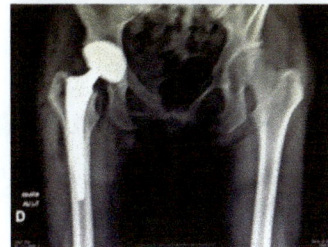

Notes:

CLUB FOOT, FEET

This is also called Congenital Talipes Equino-Varus (CTEV) which means the foot is pointing downwards and inwards. Males are more commonly affected than females at the ratio of 2:1. The calf is often smaller, the heel points inwards and upwards, and the foot points downwards with the forefoot swinging towards the midline. If untreated the child can walk, but the side of the foot then has to take the pressure of weight bearing as opposed to the sole. It is only seen now in developing countries where there is limited medical access.

TREATMENT

The aim is to get the foot in a more normal position and the sooner treatment is started the better.

Early:

Manipulative: Early treatment is to gently manipulate the foot and do this on a repeated basis and hold the position with strapping or splints or plaster casts. Later, Dennis Brown boots can be applied.

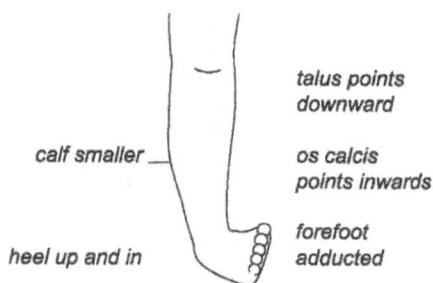

calf smaller

heel up and in

talus points downward

os calcis points inwards

forefoot adducted

Surgical: This is carried out in babies at around three months of age who have failed to respond to manipulative treatment. The ligaments on the inner side of the back of the foot are released and the tight heel cord is lengthened, ETA (Elongation Tendo Achilles).

Late:

If the child is picked up late bony fusion is necessary where the heel bone and the bone in front of it is fused together (calcaneo-cuboid fusion), usually carried out between six and nine years of age. A triple arthrodesis is where the three joints at the back of the heel are welded together.

CALCANEO-VALGUS

This is the reverse of club foot and is where the foot points outwards; usually due to the way the baby has been lying in-utero and no treatment is necessary. Sometimes manipulation is needed but mostly growth will gradually correct the problem.

Notes:

FLAT FEET (PES PLANUS)

This is due to ligamentous laxity and requires no treatment. The arch can be recreated when the child stands on tiptoes indicating normal function of the joints. Some races have naturally flat feet, such as the African races, and they are the fastest runners in the world.

Reassurance of the parents is the best treatment but sometimes insoles are required for the shoes or alteration to the heel of the shoe by lengthening the inner part of the heel. If flat feet are painful the tibialis posterior tendon on the inside of the foot can be advanced and the talo-navicular joint can be fused.

INTOEING

This is common, often associated with the squatting or frog position, and is due to increased internal rotation at the hip. Again, growth will usually correct this, and reassurance is all that is needed.

CURLY TOES

These are also very common, and they are usually in the 3rd and 4th toes where the toes are bent up excessively, but no treatment is required. Sometimes if there is pressure, a tenotomy of the tendon bending the toes down can be carried out.

KNOCK KNEES & BOWLEGS (GENU VALGUM & GENU VARUM)

This is also common particularly in children who walk early and is due to unequal development of the growth plate at the knee.

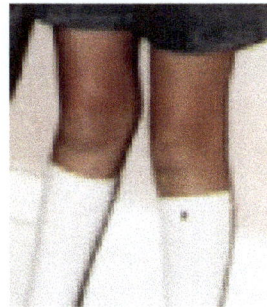

Mostly they correct as the child grows. Sometimes stapling of the growth plate at adolescence is necessary, to allow the slower growing side to catch up or, if it is a problem after growth has ceased, an osteotomy is necessary.

Notes:

SPINA BIFIDA

Because the spine develops from the ectoderm and sinks beneath the skin, occasionally this fails to complete, and a bulge develops in the lower back which is called a meningo-myelocoele or herniations of the spinal cord and coverings. This may even be open allowing drainage of the spinal fluid and is often associated with paraplegia (paralysis of the lower limbs). It is called a spina bifida overta.

Swelling of the brain due to alteration in the flow of the cerebrospinal fluid is often associated, and this is called hydrocephalus (swelling of the head).

The spinous process of the vertebra develops from either side and if they fail to meet, it is called a bifid spine and is present normally in the vertebrae of the neck (see picture of C5 spine), but abnormally in the lower back. It is called a spina bifida occulta.

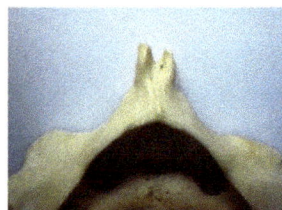

TREATMENT

1. Close defect
2. Treat paraplegia in infancy: muscle transfers or callipers
3. An ileal bladder is necessary
4. A neurosurgeon performs shunts to allow free drainage of the cerebrospinal fluid

Notes:

CEREBRAL PALSY

This occurs in about 1/1000 births and is due to brain damage from various causes such as lack of oxygen, trauma, jaundice, or infection. Brain function is usually not affected, and the child is of normal or above average intelligence.

Spastic: This is where the muscles contract uncontrollably and may produce a scissor gait or tense muscles.

Athetoid: This is where there is variation in the way the muscles contract allowing writhing movements.

TREATMENT

Treatment is by splints, muscle transfers, or tenotomies, and attendance at a normal school if the child is not grossly affected, otherwise in a special school where more nursing care is available.

MUSCLE DYSTROPHIES

This where the muscle fails to function properly, and because of paralysis of the respiratory muscles, death can occur from associated infection of the lung.

ACHONDROPLASIA

This is a condition where the normal growth of the bones is inhibited and a person develops a short stature (a dwarf) with a normal sized head, but short arms and legs and a short body.

OSTEOGENESIS IMPERFECTA

This is a condition where the bones are more fragile and is associated with collagen and calcium deficiency in bones producing brittle bones. The collagen deficiency allows the darkness of the retina to shine through such that the white in the eye appears blue.

TREATMENT

Treat fractures as they occur, and this may involve preventative treatment such as rodding of the femora and tibiae.

Notes:

OSTEOCHONDRITIS (CRUSHING, SPLITTING, PULLING)

1. CRUSHING

The blood supply to a part is cut off (tissue necrosis). The dead bone erodes and is gradually replaced (creeping substitution).

<u>Perthes Disease (hip):</u> **Georg Perthes**, 1896-1927, described this, but it was also noted by **Arthur Legg** and **Jaques Calvé**, whose names are also associated.

Ages: 5-10, boys > girls.

Symptoms: Pain, often in the knee. Limp.

Signs: "Irritable" hip. Decreased abduction of the hip.

Tests: Blood tests and x-rays are often all normal initially. X-ray change develops later with porosis and sclerosis, flattening of the head (mushroom effect) and in older patients the "sagging rope" sign.

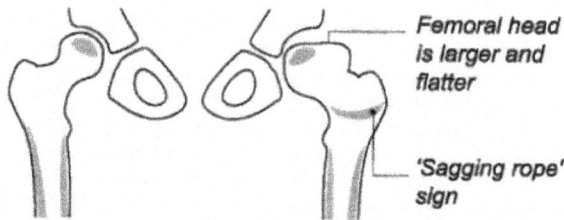

Femoral head is larger and flatter

'Sagging rope' sign

The effects depend on the amount of head of the femur involved and the age of onset. The earlier the onset and the smaller the amount of head involved, the better the prognosis.

TREATMENT

1. Bed rest for the irritable hip for two to three weeks.
2. Surgery – Innominate osteotomy to provide cover for the femoral head.

Notes:

Scheuermann's disease (spine): **Holger Scheurmann**, 1877-1960, described this in 1921.

Ages: 12-17, boys > girls.

Symptoms: Backache usually in the thoracic spine.

Signs: Increased kyphosis (adolescent kyphosis).

Tests: X-rays may show wedging of the vertebral bodies, Schmorl's nodes (disc intrusion into the bodies).

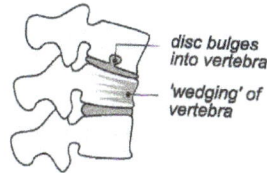

disc bulges into vertebra

'wedging' of vertebra

Christian Schmorl, 1861-1932, was Director of the Pathological Institute of Dresden, and first described these in 1932.

TREATMENT:
1. Exercises
2. Brace

2. SPLITTING

Dissecans: Part of the articular surface separates. Common in the knee, less common elbow, ankle.

Ages: 13-14, boys > girls.

Symptoms: Pain in the joint, clicking or locking.

Signs: Often normal examination.

Tests: X-rays show separate fragment or loose body.

TREATMENT

Arthroscopy and fix if possible, with wires or screws, or excise.

3. PULLING

Where a tendon pulls on an apophysis (part of the growth plate) producing inflammation (apophysitis).

Osgood-Schlatter's (knee): **Robert Osgood**, 1873-1956, and **Carl Schlatter**, 1864-1934, independently described this in 1903.

Ages: 13-15, boys > girls.

Notes:

<u>Sever's (heel):</u> **James Sever**, 1878–1964, described this.

Ages: 9-13, girls > boys.

Symptoms: Pain.

Signs: Local tenderness. Prominent tibial tubercle (knee).

Tests: X-rays sometimes show a separate ossicle in the tibial apophysis, fragmentation of the calcaneal apophysis.

This (right) is the author's adult R knee showing the separated fragment of the apophysis.

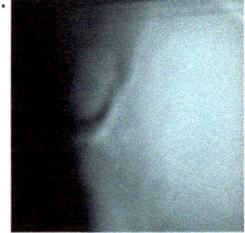

TREATMENT:

Most settle when growth ceases.

1.   Restrict activity: Football in boys (knee), ballet in girls (heel).
2.   Surgery: Excise bony fragment.

<u>Slipped Epiphysis:</u> (Sufe — Slipped Upper Femoral Epiphysis)

Ages: 10-15, boys > girls, overweight boys or tall and thin, 40% bilateral; always x-ray both hips.

a) Acute
b) Chronic

Symptoms: Pain in hip or knee, limp

Signs: The hip goes into external rotation on flexion.

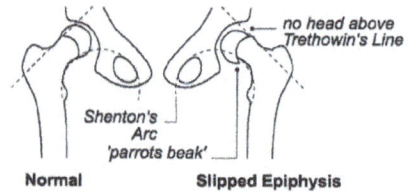

no head above Trethowin's Line

Shenton's Arc
'parrots beak'

Normal   Slipped Epiphysis

Tests: X-ray shows disordered Trethowan's line (**William Trethowan**, 1882-1934), Shenton's arc (**Edward Shenton**, 1872-1955).

TREATMENT:

Reduce if possible. Internally fix. Beware chondrolysis and early onset osteoarthritis.

Notes:

SCOLIOSIS

Deviation of the spine from the normal vertical alignment.

Cause: Idiopathic.

Ages: Commonest; female > males; teenagers.

Secondary to:

a)   neuromuscular disorders e.g., polio

b)   infection e.g., TB

c)   degeneration

Symptoms: Prominence on the back noted, often on school examination.

Signs: Lateral deviation and rotation of spine with rib hump on flexion (hunchback).

Tests: X-ray: Standing views. Angle noted in primary curve (Cobb).

TREATMENT:

Conservative:

1.   Exercises

2.   Splintage: Milwaukee brace, Risser jacket

Surgical:

Curve > 40 degrees: Spinal fusion with some form of internal fixation.

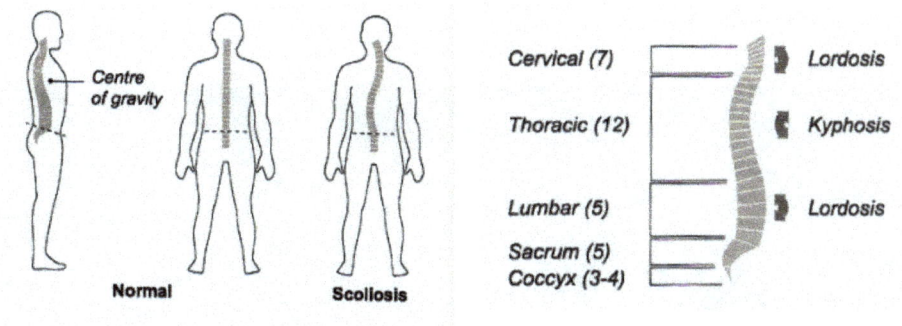

Normal   Scoliosis

Cervical (7)   Lordosis

Thoracic (12)   Kyphosis

Lumbar (5)   Lordosis

Sacrum (5)

Coccyx (3-4)

Centre of gravity

Notes:

PART TWO:

Inflammation

ACUTE OSTEOMYELITIS

This is common in young children and the bacterial infection comes via the blood stream to the growing end of the bone (metaphysis). It often does not spread into the epiphysis due to the adherence of the periosteum and cartilaginous plate of the metaphysis. It may spread into the shaft or diaphysis of the bone. Acute inflammation and pus formation follows. The pus is forced out beneath the periosteum and may spread along the shaft and around it. It may burst into the bone or out through the soft tissues. The commonest organism is Staphylococcus aureus. A loose fragment of bone is called a sequestrum and of the whole shaft an involucrum.

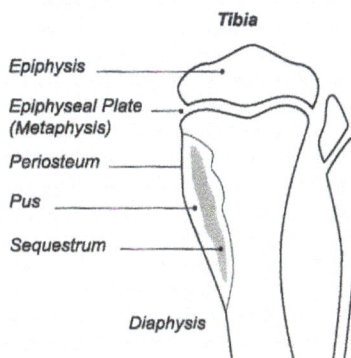

Because periosteum makes new bone when it is lifted off, a whole new shaft of the bone may form, as in the following x-rays of the author's left leg, as a baby (1939) prior to the availability of antibiotics. [Penicillin was discovered by **Alexander Fleming**, 1881-1955, in 1928, but it took **Howard Florey**, 1898-1968, and **Boris Chain**, 1906-1979, to extract a stable product in 1940, by which time World War 2 had begun.] It was treated by dressings and drained through openings in the skin over a period of six months.

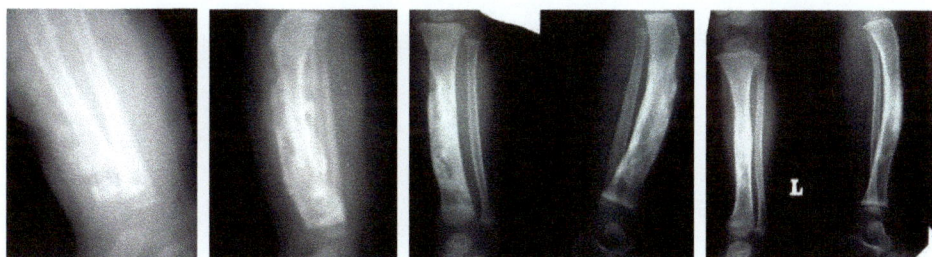

Note the new shaft developing from the initial distal involvement, the loss of the old, with a successful outcome, and normal leg length as the epiphysis was not involved.

Notes:

Symptoms: The child is ill and in acute pain.

Signs: There is fever due to septicaemia or the spread of organisms through the blood stream. Movement is possible at the joint, but the child resists movement. If there is an infection in the joint movement is not possible. This is called a septic arthritis.

Tests: Culture of the blood is taken, and a full blood screen shows a raised white count and a raised sedimentation rate. In x-rays, no changes are seen initially but later new bone is noted beneath the elevated periosteum.

TREATMENT:

Conservative:
The child is treated with bed rest and antibiotics, with broad spectrum antibiotics given initially until the offending organism is found. The affected limb is splinted.

Surgical:
Surgical treatment involves early drainage, and this may involve drilling the bone to release the pus which is often under pressure.

COMPLICATIONS AND RESULTS:
Most cases now recover fully but occasionally some go on to chronic osteomyelitis where there is recurrent infection, and this may occur even some years later. Sometimes the organisms set up a happy hunting ground in other places and form what is called metastatic abscesses. Chronic inflammation of the lining of the bone or periostitis forms and occasionally there is chronic inflammation in the muscles known as myositis.

Notes:

CHRONIC OSTEOMYELITIS

This is a chronic inflammation, usually due to an underlying sequestrum. This may be an area of bone that has lost its blood supply by acute infection, or following a fracture, or post-surgery. Sometimes the presence of a foreign body such as a screw or a joint replacement may be present, producing an irritation and further reaction and infection. Pus escapes through a sinus.

The organism is often resistant to antibiotics and the commonest organism is MRSA (Methicillin Resistant Staphylococcus Aureus). Sometimes no organism is grown especially when there has been extensive antibiotic treatment.

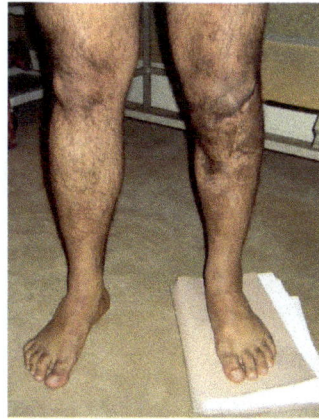

Scars tethered to bone are indications of previous osteomyelitis or healed infection. This was a complicated case with an open fracture requiring skin grafting and there was resultant shortening of the leg. He is standing on his thick file of notes which evens up the leg length discrepancy.

Symptoms: There is pain and a discharge

Signs: The skin is thickened, scaly and red and there is a sinus present with the discharge of pus.

Tests: X-ray shows the bone is thickened with osteosclerosis and porosis present. A lucent line is seen around an implant if present. Blood culture shows organisms and sensitivity.

TREATMENT:

Conservative:
The treatment is rest and antibiotics.

Surgical:
Drainage is often necessary together with irrigation and removal of the offending area of dead bone or the prosthesis. Sometimes an immediate replacement can be carried out provided there is strong antibiotic cover. If the fracture has not united it may be necessary to change to an external fixation device. The bone can be saucerised and occasionally in chronic cases with complications, amputation is considered.

Notes:

ACUTE SEPTIC ARTHRITIS

This is due to infection within the joint and the child has similar signs and symptoms to acute osteomyelitis except there is no movement possible in the joint.

TREATMENT:
The treatment is systemic antibiotics and aspiration and injection of antibiotics into the joint itself. Immediate surgical treatment is essential to prevent damage to the lining articular cartilage.

COMPLICATIONS:
If immediate treatment is not successful chondrolysis, or cartilage necrosis, may occur and arthritis develops in the joint. This is more likely if the infection becomes chronic.

POLIOMYELITIS

Unfortunately, this is still present in underdeveloped countries. It is due to a virus affecting the anterior horn cells in the spinal column producing paralysis of various muscles. It has been prevented by oral or intradermal vaccination since the 1950s and is rarely found in developed countries now. The consequences are due to the weakness of muscles. Like smallpox, eradicated in 1977, it is hoped to be eradicated this decade.

Muscle strength is assessed by the following scale:

0. Total paralysis
1. Flicker
2. Contraction but not strong enough to overcome gravity
3. Strong enough to overcome gravity
4. Strong but not normal
5. Normal

Child Affected:
The growth is retarded, the limb is shortened and thin and there is atrophic skin and thin bones.

TREATMENT
Conservative:
Splintage: Callipers, built up shoe.

Notes:

Surgical:

a) Leg lengthening
b) Tendon transfers
c) Joint fusion if there is a dropped foot

TUBERCULOSIS

This, again, is uncommon in developed countries but common in developing countries. Unfortunately, the organism of the tubercle bacillus has become resistant to antibiotics and is now recurrent particularly in the lower socio-economic groups who fail to finish their course of treatment or get lost to follow up. The bacillus infects the lung and the lymph nodes and is spread to the bones and joints by the blood stream. It can be prevented by the BCG vaccination. It used to be common in infected dairy herds producing infected milk.

General effect: Night sweats and weight loss.

Local effects: The joint is usually swollen and there is associated muscle wasting and stiffness.

There is increased kyphosis in the spine, called a kyphus, when a vertebra collapses. It used to be called Pott's disease, described by **Percival Pott**, 1714-1788, in 1758, or spinal tuberculosis.

TREATMENT:
Conservative:
Drugs: Rifampicin, Isoniazid, Ethambutol, Streptomycin, Pyrazinamide.
Surgical:
Drain the abscess or irrigate the joint and remove the synovial membrane.

COMPLICATIONS:
Stiffness in the joint due to scarring, sinus formation, and late recurrence.

Notes:

PART THREE:

Traumatic Orthopaedics

FRACTURES AND DISLOCATIONS

The cause is a force either applied directly or indirectly. The degree of damage depends on the amount of force applied and the resilience of the tissues.

Bone is a hard tissue, and a fracture is a break in a bone. There is also damage to soft tissues such as bruising, haematoma, or laceration and grazing of the skin. A sprain is a stretching of the ligaments, a subluxation is a joint partially out of socket where the capsule is torn, and a dislocation is where the joint is fully out of socket.

Pathological fractures may occur with minimal force indicating underlying disease such as osteoporosis or metastatic deposits from carcinoma or sarcoma.

Stress (fatigue) fractures occur following repetitive minor force and are commonly called shin splints in the leg, or march fractures in the foot.

Types:

1. Closed or open with perforation of the overlying soft tissues from within or without
2. Simple or complicated involving vessels and nerves. There is always soft tissue damage associated and this affects the outcome

They are classified according to the appearance of the bone ends at the fracture site and fracture description relates to the distal fragment (angulation or rotation). Various classifications are used.

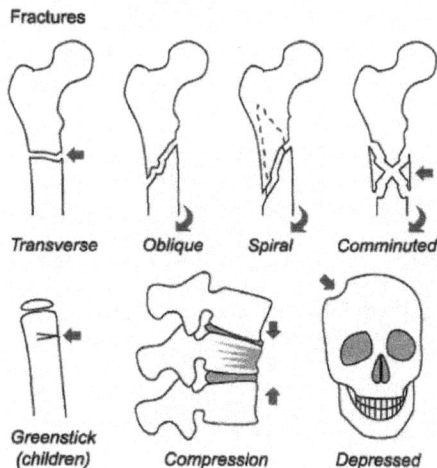

Fractures

Transverse   Oblique   Spiral   Comminuted

Greenstick (children)   Compression   Depressed

Notes:

Symptoms: Pain and loss of function.

Signs: Are the same as for inflammation with deformity, swelling, bruising and tenderness and often crepitus at the fracture site.

Tests: Involves x-rays, MRI, CT scans, and ultrasound.

TREATMENT:

Aim: Complete and early restoration of function. Before treatment can be considered it is important to know:

Site: Where the fracture is, i.e., at the end or middle.

Types: The type of fracture.

Displacement: Seen on x-ray on two views, AP and lateral, e.g., impacted, angulated, rotated, displaced. Remember the description relates to the distal fragment.

General:

1. First aid and transport to the hospital or surgery
2. Pain relief
3. Blood replacement if necessary

Local: 'Reduce, hold, use.

REDUCE:

Restore to correct alignment by:

a) Closed manipulation which is the art of orthopaedics or good bone setting which orthopaedic surgeons used to be called (bone setters).

b) Open reduction (if closed impossible or inaccurate).

c) Not all fractures require reduction and a poor position in children can be accepted as growth will correct the deformity, but not rotational deformity as shown in the following pictures. The child was an 8-year-old girl who had fallen from a tree.

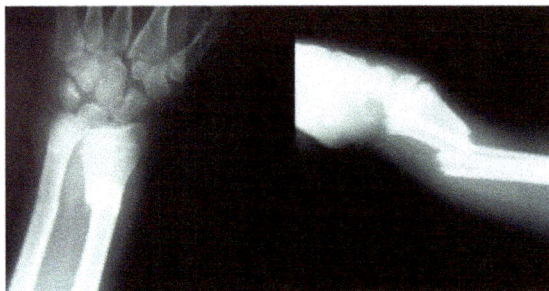

Note the forearm is bent, but the alignment is good although the fracture is displaced.

Notes:

After two attempts at closed reduction the forearm is straight, but the radius is still displaced.

Unfortunately, young surgeons find it difficult to resist operating on such a fracture.

There are only two fractures in children that demand open reduction, and these are fractures of the lateral epicondyle in the elbow and fractures of the surgical neck of the femur.

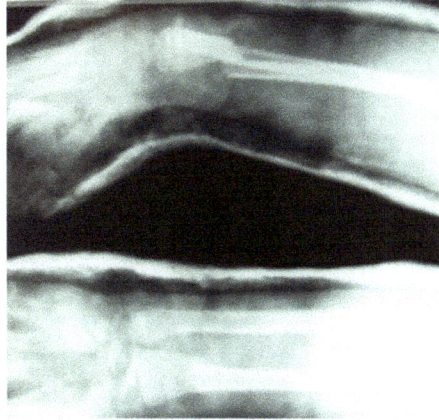

Six weeks later and union has occurred. Note the spread of new bone from the lifting of the periosteum. Remodelling will occur.

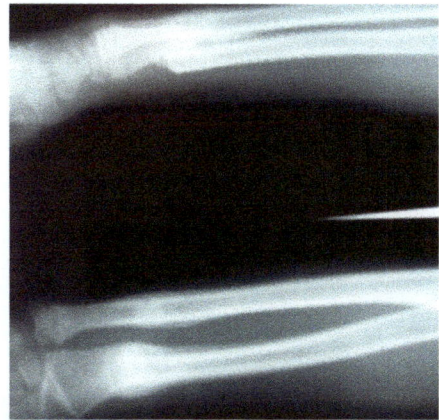

By one year it is difficult to see where the bone has been broken.

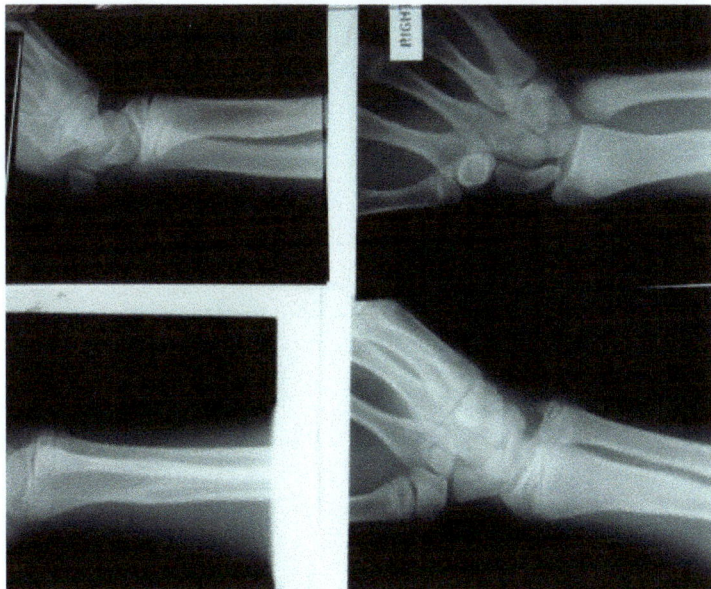

HOLD:

This is only necessary if the fracture is unstable, or potentially unstable.

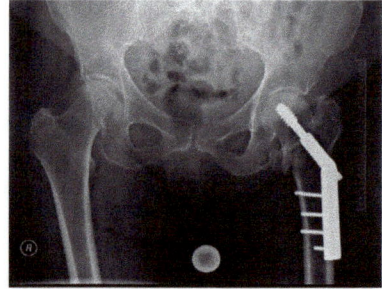

1. By plaster of paris (POP) or plastic, splintage or traction..

2. By internal fixation with screws, wires, pins and nails, and again one has to be aware of the pitfalls of surgery. ORIF (Open Reduction Internal Fixation).

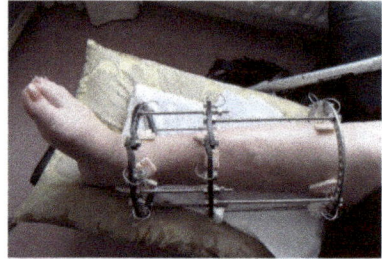

3. A combination such as the use of an external fixator, first pioneered by **Gavril Ilazarov,** 1921–1992, and this is particularly useful in open fractures.

USE:

The most important aspect of treatment is to maintain and restore function. It involves exercising muscles and joints not immobilised with the aid of physiotherapy.

Note the knee bending even with the fixator in place.

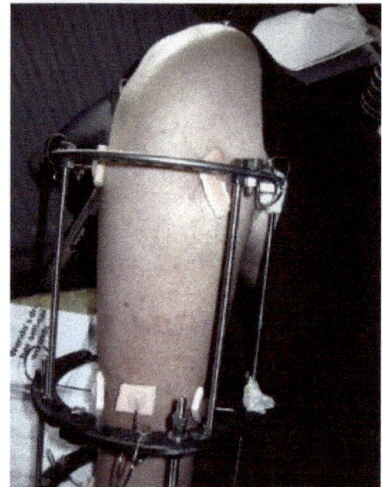

Notes:

HEALING OF FRACTURES/TISSUES

Healing is progressive and commences immediately. A good blood supply is essential for proper healing. It is divided into stages but is a continuous process.

Stage 1

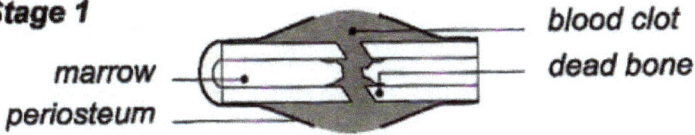

blood clot

marrow

dead bone

periosteum

Haematoma: As bone bleeds a clot (haematoma) forms between the broken ends. Bruising and swelling may be seen.

Stage 2

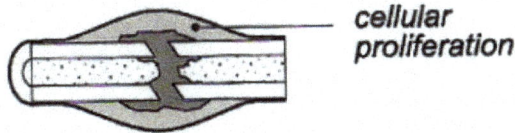

cellular proliferation

Cellular proliferation: Fibroblasts, chondroblasts, osteoblasts and macrophages invade the haematoma over the succeeding 10 days. An increased blood supply is established.

Stage 3

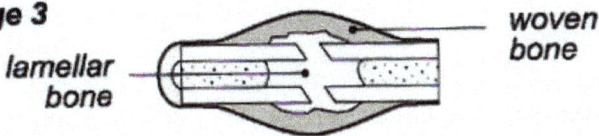

woven bone

lamellar bone

Callus: Woven bone is formed, and calcification starts to occur over the next four-six weeks allowing the fracture to become firm.

Stage 4

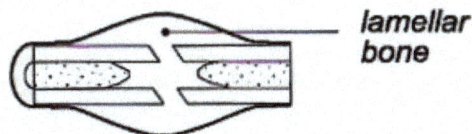

lamellar bone

Consolidation: Lamella bone is formed and bone is laid down in lines of stress. This takes several months. Clinical union occurs during this phase.

Notes:

Stage 5

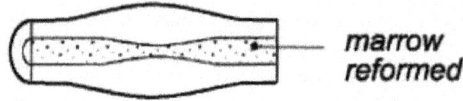

marrow
reformed

Remodelling: The bone is restored as nearly as possible to the original and this process can take up to two years.

Direct healing is seen in rigid internal fixation with no obvious callus. Indirect healing where there is some movement at the fracture ends shows callus.

Clinical union is defined when the bone is stable on examination. Radiological union is defined when the fracture is consolidated on x-ray. MRI scans unfortunately are often misinterpreted as showing non-union of a fracture when there is both clinical and radiological union, due to the amount of water present at the fracture site.

Time: Children get half price, so they get half the time.

	Spiral Fracture	Transverse
Upper Limb	6 weeks	12 weeks
Lower Limb	12 weeks	24 weeks

FACTORS AFFECTING HEALING:

There are various factors that can affect healing including the age of the patient and their general health. The local effects are:

1. Degree of local trauma
2. Degree of bone loss
3. Type of bone (compact, cancellous)
4. Degree of stability
5. Infection
6. Involvement of joint (synovial fluid)
7. Presence of local malignancy
8. Radiation necrosis

Notes:

COMPLICATIONS:

General:

1. Shock, due to loss of blood and fluids, or hypovolaemia. Treatment is with fluid and blood replacement.

2. Crush syndrome, where muscles are destroyed and release a toxin resulting in renal failure. It occurs commonly with fallen masonry and earthquakes.

3. Treatment is to resect the muscles, or even amputation, and kidney dialysis.

4. Fat embolism. This occurs with long bone fractures and is due to the release of fatty acids into the blood stream setting up an inflammation of the lung or pneumonitis. It occurs in the first few days following injury. Hypoxia results in increased respiratory rate, increased heart rate, and cerebral confusion. Petechial haemorrhages, or tiny little spots of blood, can be seen in the skin or in the eyes.

   Test: blood gases show low arterial oxygen. Sometimes there is an elevated temperature. Treatment is with oxygen and steroids, sometimes with a respirator, IPPR (Intermittent Positive Pressure Respiration).

5. Deep Vein Thrombosis (DVT) and Pulmonary Embolism (PE). This occurs when there is sluggish circulation through the veins allowing clots to form in the deep veins. Breaking from these clots travelling to the lungs causes pulmonary embolism and can be fatal.

   Treatment is best by prophylaxis with exercises, elevation of the limbs and low molecular weight heparin. Once the condition has been diagnosed, it is necessary to anti-coagulate the patient with heparin and warfarin.

Local:

1. **Bone**

   a) *Delayed union*: This is due to a poor blood supply with a large gap and excessive movement and infection. It is common in tubular bones where there is thick cortex and little cancellous bone such as the clavicle and tibia.

   b) *Non-union*: Occurs where the callus is replaced by fibrous or scar tissue (pseudarthrosis). Treatment of delayed and non-union is by

Notes:

electrical stimulation, high frequency sound waves or lithotripsy, and bone grafting, bringing in bone cells from, for example, the pelvic crest. Sometimes all that is necessary is to freshen the bone ends and internally fix a fracture. If there are screws used in rods, for example in the tibia, the top or bottom screws can be removed to allow the bone to slide along the rod (dynamisation).

c) *Mal-union*: This occurs when the fracture is allowed to join in a faulty position either by inadequate reduction or fixation. It can sometimes be accepted but otherwise is treated by osteotomy. Shortening may occur.

d) *Avascular necrosis*: This occurs when the blood supply is interrupted particularly in the neck of the femur or the waist of the scaphoid.

e) *Osteoporosis*: This is due to disuse and patients must be encouraged to weight bear if possible and undertake an exercise programme. Sometimes a condition called Complex Regional Pain Syndrome may occur where this is alteration in the blood supply producing pain and skin sensation changes.

f) *Prominent metal ware*: This is seen when a plate and screws, for example, is used to fix a clavicle fracture and the screw heads become prominent requiring removal once the fracture has joined.

2. **Joint**

Stiffness is the commonest complication usually due to prolonged immobilisation, and lack of exercise in the joints not immobilised. Once it develops, it is treated by physiotherapy and sometimes manipulation under anaesthetic.

It is best prevented by encouraging exercise from the beginning. The patient must be reassured that they will do no harm and to move even if it hurts.

Osteoarthritis occurs when the joint surface has been damaged.

3. **Soft tissue damage**

Soft tissues are always involved in fractures and sometimes specific damage occur to, for example, nerves in some situations such as a humeral fracture involving the radial nerve or vessels such as the popliteal artery behind the knee, or muscles. These become wasted due to disuse.

Notes:

There is a condition called the Compartment Syndrome where swelling in the muscles affects the blood supply producing intense pain. It is diagnosed by measuring the compartmental pressure and the treatment is by emergency fasciotomy. The late result is scarring in the muscle producing contracture such as Volkmann's contracture, (**Richard Volkmann**, 1830-1889) or clawing of the hand or foot.

4. **Infection**

    This is common following open fractures or surgery, and the treatment is as for osteomyelitis, with antibiotics and wound debridement.

FRACTURES AND DISLOCATIONS IN THE UPPER LIMB

Function is important: Do not immobilise too long.

Fractured clavicle: Very common. Union good. 'Figure 8' for three weeks or sling only. Warn mother of lump of callus in a child.

Dislocation Acromio-clavicular (AC) joint:

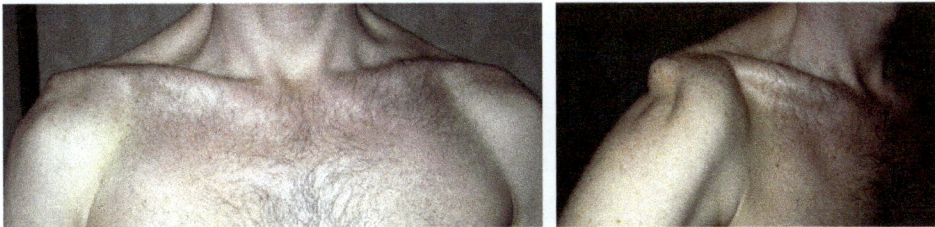

Internal fixation plate needs removal three-six months later. The x-rays are from a different patient. If left alone, function is often normal, despite deformity

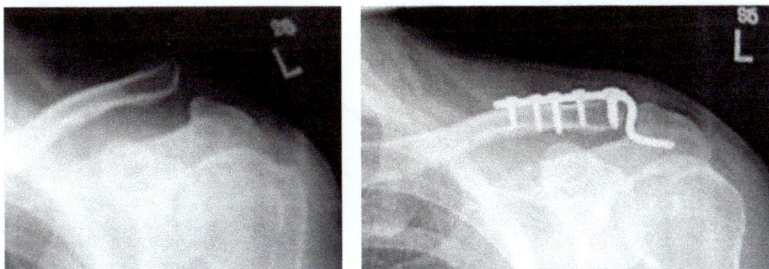

Notes:

Fractured scapula: Sling for a few days.

Fractured neck of humerus: Common. Elderly patients. Impacted fracture. Sling for two weeks under clothes then exercise.

Dislocated shoulder: Common anterior.

> *Reduce*: Kocher manoeuvre (traction, externally rotate, adduct, internally rotate). Hippocratic (foot in axilla, pull and adduct).
>
> *Hold*: Sling/body bandage three-six weeks.
>
> *Use*: Exercises.

Recurrent dislocation: Common, requires surgery, fix detached labrum from glenoid (socket).

Fracture shaft humerus: Collar and cuff sling and gravity. POP splints. ORIF often needed. Beware radial nerve damage (it passes in a groove diagonally from front to back in the midshaft).

Supracondylar: Common in children. Always admit; watch for arterial damage. Gross swelling. If necessary, traction in extension. Mal-union produces gunstock deformity.

Fractured neck & head of radius: Excise if comminuted. Exercise.

Fractured olecranon: Gap fracture, reduce, – hold by internal fixation (e.g., tension band wiring).

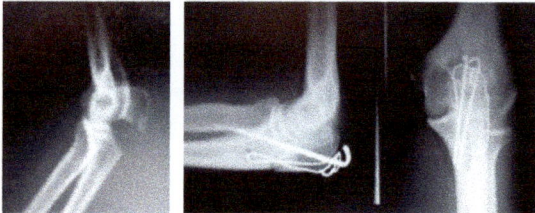

Dislocated elbow: Reduce. Stable. Sling for few days.

Fractured radius & ulna (both bones): Difficult to hold, often best to operate.

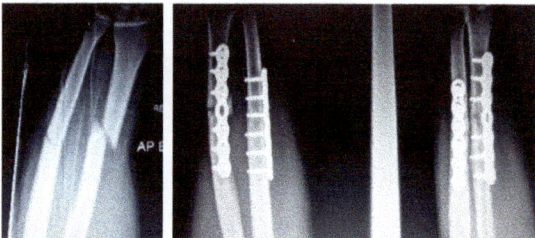

Notes:

Fractured radius & dislocated ulna: At wrist – **Ricardo Galliazzi**, 1866-1952.

Fractured ulna & dislocated radius: At elbow – **Giovanni Monteggia**, 1762-1815.

Always make sure both elbow and wrist joints are included in the x-ray if there is a single bone fracture. Open reduction nearly always necessary.

Colles fracture: This was first described by **Abraham Colles,** 1773-1843, in 1814 which he did without the benefit of x-rays. Very common. Fall on an outstretched hand.

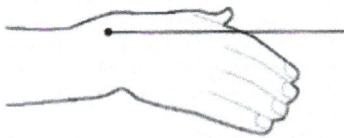

Dinner Fork Deformity (Radial deviation, dorsal displacement, backward angulation, comminution)

Reduce: Traction on thumb and index finger, pronate, ventrally displace.

Hold: POP cast four-six weeks. Re x-ray in one week as often re-displaces.

N.B. Advise exercises. Shoulder, elbow, and fingers.

Smith's fracture/Barton's fracture: **Robert Smith** 1807-1873, **John Barton** 1794-1871. Reversed Colles. May require open reduction and fixation with buttress plate.

Fractured scaphoid: Common. Blood supply may be affected. If suspected (tender anatomical snuffbox) POP cast, re x-ray one week, 10 days. Cast six-eight weeks, may require screw fixation.

Dislocation of wrist (lunate): Often missed. CT scan if unsure. Open reduction often necessary.

Fractured metacarpals: Usually no fixation. Exercise fingers.

Fractured base 1st metacarpal: **Edward Bennett's** (1837-1907) fracture. Abduct thumb, may require open reduction.

Skier's, biker's thumb: This used to be called gamekeeper's thumb. It is a rupture of the ligament on the inner side of the metacarpo-phalangeal joint due to forced abduction of the thumb. Often needs repair.

Notes:

Fractured neck 5th metacarpal: Boxer's fracture. Difficult to hold, not reduced, exercise fingers. Leaves a deformity but no loss of function.

Fractured phalanges: Strap to adjacent finger.

PIP (Proximal Inter-phalangeal) dislocation: Commonly seen in cricketers where the ball strikes the outstretched finger. Reduce. Exercise.

Mallet finger: Rupture extensor tendon or base of distal phalanx. Splint six weeks. Occasionally repair tendon.

FRACTURES AND SPRAINS OF THE SPINE

Spinal injuries may be:
1.   Stable
2.   Unstable – beware spinal cord damage.

Mechanism of injury:
Falls. Sport (rugby). Lifting. Motor Vehicle Accidents (MVA). Falling masonry (bombs, earthquakes).

Types:
1.   **Extension:** Chip fracture off anterior longitudinal ligament (avulsion fractures)
2.   **Flexion:** Crush or wedge compression fracture
3.   **Compression:** Straight spine, burst fracture
4.   **Rotation:** Plus combination of flexion
     •   unstable – may produce dislocation of facet joints
     •   unstable – spinal cord at risk

STABLE FRACTURES AND SPRAINS

CERVICAL SPINE
1.   Soft tissue injury or muscular ligamentous sprain
     This is common following rear impact motor vehicle accidents and whiplash is a term commonly used. (It was first used by **Harold Crowe**, 1895-1989[?], at a conference in 1928.) It is more the mechanism of injury, which is a backward and forward jolt of the head on the neck. The backward movement of the head is now prevented by the headrest and the forward movement by the chin hitting the chest.

Notes:

Since sash belts have been introduced, whiplash injuries have become more common.

In a rear shunt the vehicle that is struck is called the target vehicle, and the striking vehicle a bullet vehicle. Because the bullet vehicle is at fault legally, it is interesting to note that the victims of the target vehicle are the ones that develop symptoms whereas the mechanism of injury is the same. It is similarly noted that when cars are stationary, and somebody reverses into a target vehicle, again it is the victim that complains of symptoms.

Litigation has been shown to prolong symptoms and often they do not resolve after completion of the case. The muscles most involved are the muscles in the back of the neck, but sometimes also in drivers the muscles of the rotator cuff can be involved producing pain in lifting the arm from the side. Airbags were invented to prevent forward jolting of the body as Americans objected to wearing seatbelts. Symptoms develop even in low velocity accidents. Avoid over-treatment.

2. **Wedge, crush, or compression fractures**

    Symptoms:

    - Pain; neck, back of shoulder (trapezius)
    - Down arm (brachialgia)
    - Headache
    - Stiffness

    Signs: Restricted movements. Wry neck.

    Tests:

    - X-ray – often normal or may show loss of lordosis in sprains. Wedge shaped vertebra in fractures.
    - MRI – may show disc lesion, but often present in normal population as degeneration commences in the 20s and increases linearly with age. It is not necessarily symptomatic. Almost always at C5/6.
    - CT – in presence of fracture to determine if cord threatened.
    - EMG – assess peripheral nerves in arm.

Notes:

TREATMENT:

General:

1. Analgesics or painkillers
2. Anti-inflammatory (particularly slow-release) drugs
3. Relaxants such as diazepam in the first two weeks or in chronic symptoms amitriptyline, a mild tranquillizer that is taken at night.

Local:

1. A collar is often useful for the first one-two weeks although exercise is more commonly recommended now. A soft pillow is helpful.
2. Physiotherapy – traction, ultrasound, short wave diathermy, TENS machine (Transcutaneous Electrical Nerve Stimulation), hydrotherapy, massage
3. Exercises such as swimming, cycling, rowing, exercise at a gym, Pilates, yoga, walking, dancing, and posture all help
4. Manipulation with or without anaesthetic
5. Chiropractic
6. Osteopathy
7. Acupuncture
8. Alternative therapy e.g., Aromatherapy, Naturopathy, Bowen, Reflexology, Hypnotherapy
9. Trigger point injections, facet joint injections often under the supervision of a pain clinic

The majority of patients with neck sprains recover within six months, but recovery can take as long as three years, and some are left with permanent symptoms. Studies have shown no acceleration of spondylosis or degenerative change, which renders the spine more susceptible to a spraining injury.

Notes:

THORACIC/LUMBAR SPINE

Low back sprain:
Soft tissue injury, muscular ligamentous sprain, facet joint sprain. Usually after heavy lifting. (Disc injury, see Spinal Disorders page 103).

Compression fracture:
Wedge, crush. Usually after fall, spontaneous in elderly osteoporotic women.

Symptoms: Pain, Stiffness.

Signs: Reduced movement, especially flexion. Kyphus, (a prominent angle in the spine), Dowager hump (increased forward bend in old women in the thoracic spine).

Tests:
*   X-ray – Loss of lordosis in sprains. Wedging of anterior vertebra in fractures, as shown here, in the author's old Lumbar 1 vertebral fracture with associated degeneration

*   Generalised osteoporosis

*   Osteolysis (metastatic deposit)

*   Blood – Acid phosphatase if prostatic secondary suspected (raised); Alkaline phosphatase if lung, breast secondary suspected (raised)

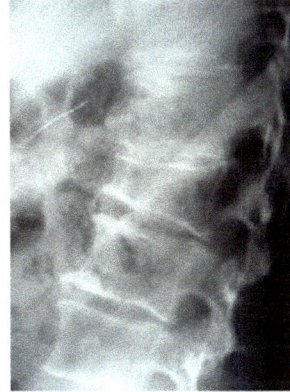

TREATMENT:

General:
1.   Bed rest
2.   Fracture board
3.   Drugs; analgesics, anti-inflammatories, relaxants

Local:
1.   Corset, brace, plaster jacket
2.   Physiotherapy
3.   Exercises, swimming

Complications:
1.   Urinary retention
2.   Constipation
3.   Stiffness, may need manipulation

SPONDYLOLYSIS

Defect in the pedicle or pars interarticularis ('collar'). Often asymptomatic. Nearly all at lumbo-sacral junction.

Tests: X-ray – oblique – Scotty dog; collar.

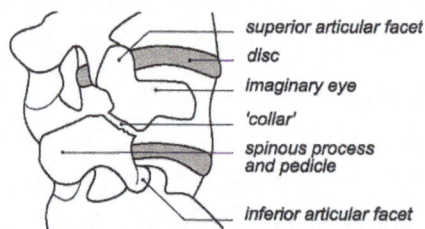

'Scotty Dog' (oblique view)

- superior articular facet
- disc
- imaginary eye
- 'collar'
- spinous process and pedicle
- inferior articular facet

SPONDYLOLISTHESIS

Seen in 5% of the population. Grade 1 (a little as in x-ray shown)-Grade 4 (almost complete) forward displacement of vertebra. A sulcus (depression) may be present in low back.

Sometimes back pain +/- sciatica.

Treatment: Brace, exercises, and physiotherapy; spinal fusion if severe and symptomatic.

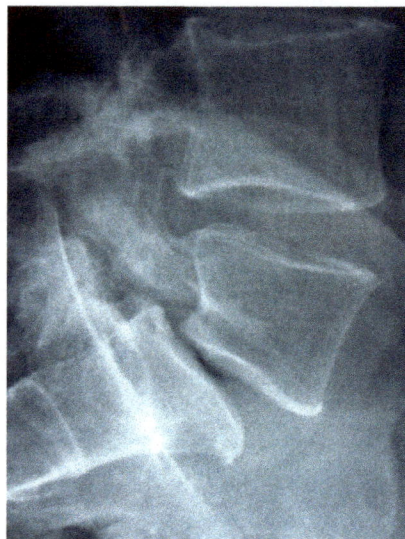

Notes:

UNSTABLE FRACTURES AND FRACTURE DISLOCATIONS

CERVICAL, THORACIC, LUMBAR SPINES

Immediate management is very important to end result.

1. Transport to Spinal Injuries Unit without delay
2. Take care to avoid further injury. Stabilise spine until properly assessed: hard collar. Spinal board
3. Maintain airway and ventilation

Cord damage:
In 40% of cervical fractures, 5% thoracic/lumbar.

Lateral cervical spine x-ray (all seven and T1) mandatory in all patients sustaining an injury above the clavicle.

Signs:
1. Spinal shock: Loss of sensation. Loss of reflexes
2. Return of muscle function and spasms, rigidity (days to weeks later)

Quadriplegia: Paralysis all four limbs (**Christopher Reeve** 1952-2004, Superman)

Paraplegia: Paralysis lower limbs.

Hemiplegia: Paralysis of one side of the body (due to cerebrovascular accident/stroke).

TREATMENT:
- Reduce: Open reduction if necessary
- Hold: Skull traction (Crutchfield tongs) in C spine. Spinal fusion
- Good nursing: Essential. Applies to any patient especially the elderly.

a) **Skin:**
Anaesthetic skin develops pressure sores within hours
- No creases in sheets; no crumbs in bed
- Two-hourly turning
- Wash and dry skin carefully
- Use powder and oil
- Adjust pillows
- Spinal beds – ripple mattresses
- Turning beds, moving patient helped if spine fused

....

Notes:

b) **Bladder:**

Avoid infection (ultimately leads to renal failure and death)

- Catheterisation – strict asepsis
- Change weekly
- Antiseptics, antibiotics
- Train bladder by filling and emptying

c) **Bowel:**

Avoid constipation

- Train by aperients, enemas
- Abdominal exercises

d) **Muscles and joints:**

Avoid contractures

- Physiotherapy
- Passive stretching

e) **Morale:**

Avoid depression

- Find role models
- Occupational Therapy
- Specialty workshops
- Sports (Paralympics).

Notes:

FRACTURES OF THE PELVIS

Pelvic Ring Fractures:

Displacement slight. Complications rare.

TREATMENT:

- Rest, analgesics, mobilise when pain allows

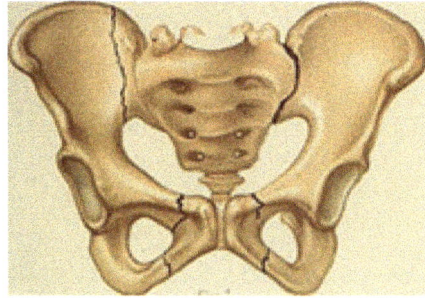

Pelvic Ring Disruptions:

Displacement severe, large blood loss.

Complications common:

- Genito-urinary tears
- Iliac vessel tears

TREATMENT:

- Reduce: Traction, open reduction and fixation
- Repair: Soft tissue injury
  - Combined surgical approach depends on tissue damage

Avulsion Fractures:

TREATMENT:

- Mobilise when comfortable

Sacrococcygeal Injuries:

Coccydynia (painful tailbone)

TREATMENT:

- Avoid sitting in acute phase, ring cushion
- Injection of local anaesthetic and steroid.
- Excise coccyx (coccygectomy, results variable)

Notes:

FRACTURES AND DISLOCATIONS IN LOWER LIMB

1. **Fractures In Femoral Neck:**
    a) Sub-capital (intracapsular), 60-70 age group
    b) Inter-trochanteric (extracapsular), 70-80 age group. More common in females as they outlive men.
    c) Sub-trochanteric

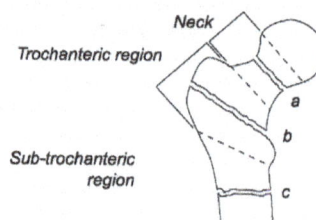

Signs: Leg short, externally rotated

Important queries as they affect length of stay:
a) Could patient walk before?
b) Home circumstances. Activities of Daily Living (ADL)?
c) Mental state

In general, patient moves down i.e., if independent, goes to live with relative; if there already, goes to a nursing home.

TREATMENT:

*   **Reduce:** All require operation, and as patient is often frail, operate as soon as possible
*   **Hold:**
a) Range is Garden type 1 (minor displacement) to 4 (total displacement). (**Robert Garden**, 1910-1982.)

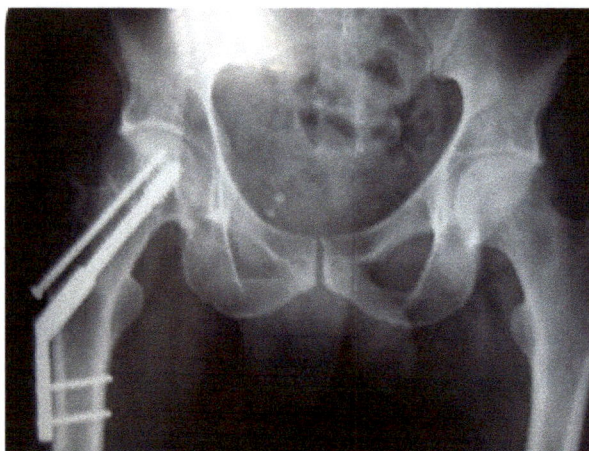

1-2 (mild): Internal fixation with compression screws

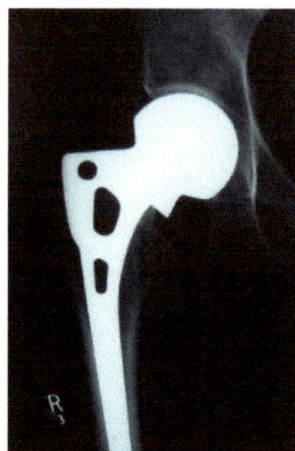

3-4 (severe): Replace femoral head (Moore's, Thompson's prosthesis, or total hip)

b) Inter-trochanteric: Dynamic Hip Screw (DHS)

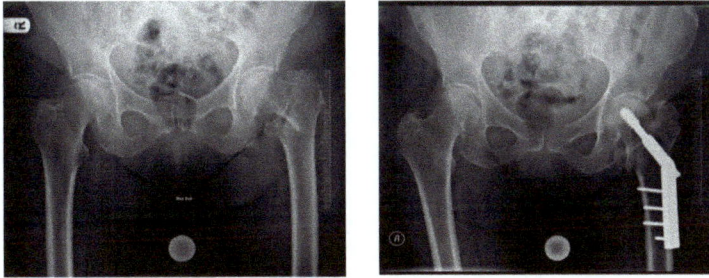

c) Sub-trochanteric: Intramedullary rod e.g., Russell Taylor nail.

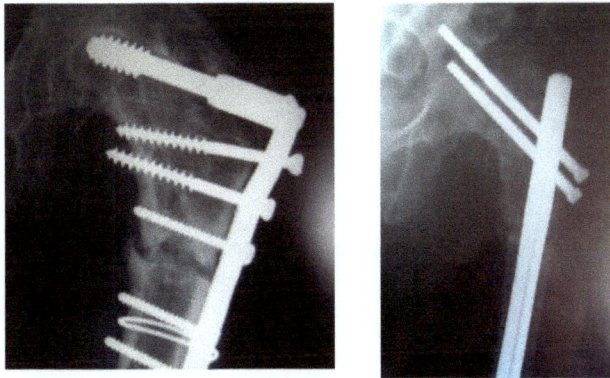

This was a difficult fracture as the hip was previously fused, and the initial plate and screws failed requiring the subsequent revision to an intra-medullary nail.

Use: Commence walking as soon as possible.

Complications:
1. Delayed union, non-union
2. Avascular necrosis (30% Garden 3-4 therefore primary replacement)
3. DVT and pulmonary embolism
4. 50% of patients die within two years because they are old and have concomitant disease

Notes:

2. **Dislocation of Hip Joint**
   - Posterior common, blow on knee. Hip flexed, leg adducted, internally rotated, but beware concomitant fracture shaft when leg lies in external rotation.
   - Anterior. Leg abducted externally rotated.
   - Medial. Fracture pelvis (floor of acetabulum).

   TREATMENT
   - Reduce: Under general anaesthetic by manipulation, open reduction and internal fixation, if associated pelvic fracture
   - Hold: By traction
   - Use: Exercise

3. **Femoral Shaft Fracture:**
   1-2 litre blood loss, fractures may be high, low.
   a) Transverse
   b) Oblique
   c) Comminuted

   TREATMENT:
   Conservative:
   - Traction: Skin, skeletal pin through proximal tibia, ropes, pulleys and weights. Various: Perkins, Hamilton Russell, Thomas splint

   Operative:
   - Intramedullary nailing under image intensifier control, with interlocking screws.

4. **Fractures into Knee Joint**
   Aspirate haemarthrosis. Accurate reduction. Internal fixation. Beware popliteal artery damage; vascular surgeon on hand, or transfer to centre with vascular unit.

5. **Patella Fractures**
   a) Intact extensor mechanism (no gap). Aspirate haemarthrosis, minimal support, active exercises
   b) Displaced. Open reduction and tension band wiring. Patellectomy if comminuted (repair extensor quadriceps mechanism)

Notes:

6. **Ligament Tears**

   Medial, lateral, cruciate – increased "play", positive drawer sign. MRI helpful.

   TREATMENT

   Conservative: Aspirate haemarthrosis, cast or splint, physiotherapy

   Surgical:

   a) Open repair medial or lateral
   b) Late reconstruction Anterior Cruciate Ligament (ACL)

7. **Recurrent Dislocation Patella**

   Common in teenage girls. Lateral dislocation (altered anatomical slope), lax ligaments.

   TREATMENT:

   Conservative: Strengthen quadriceps

   Surgical: Re-align patellar tendon

8. **Tibial Fractures**

   Proximal, middle, lower third.

   a) Transverse
   b) Spiral or oblique
   c) Comminuted
   d) Fatigue or stress (shin splints)

   High ratio cortical bone therefore delayed, non-union likely. Beware compartment syndrome – fasciotomy all four.

   TREATMENT

   Conservative:

   - Reduce: Manipulation under GA
   - Hold: Plaster or fibre cast
   - Use: Crutches non or partial weight bearing (NWB, PWB)

   Surgical: Elevation on Braun frame with calcaneal pin traction to reduce swelling for two weeks if comminuted, and very swollen. Intramedullary nailing with proximal and distal locking screws. Reamed nailing promotes osteoblastic activity.

Notes:

9. Ankle

a) Sprains. Lateral ligament common. If total tear suspected - stress inversion x-ray, or MRI. May require open repair.

TREATMENT:
- Ice, strapping, physiotherapy

b) Fractures. Inversion and eversion with rotation. Medical and/or lateral and/or posterior malleoli. Various classifications (used to be called Pott's fractures after **Percival Pott,** 1714 to 1788, who wrote numerous articles whilst laid up following an open fracture of his leg when he was thrown from his horse in 1758. His son-in-law wrote:

Conscious of the dangers attendant on fractures of this nature and thoroughly aware how much they may be increased by rough treatment or improper position he would not suffer himself to be moved until he had made the necessary disposition.

He sent to Westminster for two chairmen to bring their poles; the patient lay on the cold pavement, it being the middle of January until they arrived. In this situation he purchased a door to which he made them nail their poles. When all was ready, he caused himself to be laid on it, and was carried home.

He was examined by his fellow surgeons and although many wanted to carry out an amputation it was decided to treat it conservatively. He retained his leg and, whilst laid up, wrote many articles including the management of his fracture [see also TB p 67].

TREATMENT:
Conservative:
- Reduce: Manipulation
- Hold: Below knee cast four-six weeks
- Use: Crutches

Surgical:
Fix lateral side with plate and screws, medial, posterior with cancellous screws.

Notes:

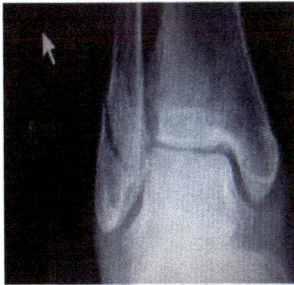 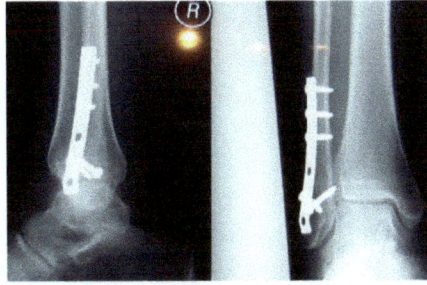

Right ankle

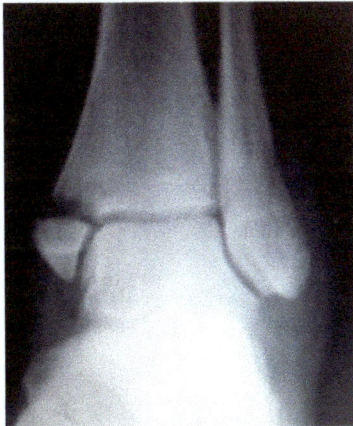 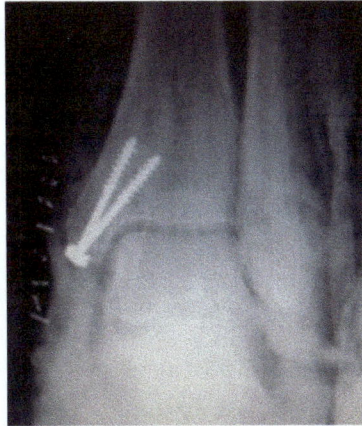

Left ankle

10. Fractures of Talus/Calcaneus

Fractures of the neck of the talus may jeopardise the blood supply and accurate reduction necessary.

TREATMENT
Conservative: Ice, elevation, compression bandage, crutches (non-weight bearing) two months.
Surgical: Internal fixation. Arthrodese subtalar joint if pain persists.

11. Fractured Metatarsals

a) Base of 5th. Common. Crepe bandage, crutches, sometimes screw fixation.

b) Neck of 3rd. (March or stress fracture). Often noted on x-ray with callus present.

12. Fractured Toes

Aspirate subungual haematoma. Strap to adjacent toe.

Notes:

PERIPHERAL NERVE LESIONS

Nerves are like fibre optic cables that transmit impulses to and from the brain via relay junctions in the spinal cord. They consist of fibres or axons collected into bundles surrounded by a sheath.

Damage may be a complete division of a nerve known as a neurotmesis, or incomplete division with disrupted axons within the sheath called axonotmesis, or bruising of the nerve called neuropraxia where the impulses are unable to be transmitted but the nerve is intact.

Following division, bleeding occurs at the nerve ends and a clot forms into which grow the axons from the proximal end whilst the distal end degenerates. If the axons are interrupted or obstructed a neuroma will form. The growth is usually 1-2mm a day. The distal end of the nerve degenerates and this is known as Wallerian degeneration.

Clinical features depend on the nerve that is damaged; whether it is mixed carrying both motor and sensory fibres or just sensory fibres in which case the area supplied is numb.

Treatment involves repair if there has been division of a nerve which can be immediate or delayed. If the gap is too large a nerve graft may be used with an operating microscope and fine materials.

With an axonotmesis or neuropraxia a 'wait-and-see' approach is adopted.

Multiple nerve injuries, such as a brachial plexus lesion in the neck, is difficult to treat, or a large nerve such as the median or sciatic nerve.

Late treatment may involve tenotomy if muscles are contracted, or tendon transfers for example, transferring the tibialis posterior from behind the leg into the tibialis anterior on the front of the leg correcting drop foot deformity.

Notes:

MUSCLE AND TENDON INJURIES

When a muscle contracts violently it can overcome its tensile strength, producing a tear within the muscle itself or a tear of the tendon. It is commonly seen in the hamstrings of athletes or footballers, occasionally in the rectus femoris where it attaches to the upper pole of the patella (kneecap) with the patient unable to straight-leg raise his foot from the bed. It requires repair.

1. **Achilles Tendon**

    A common injury is an Achilles tendon rupture which is felt as a sharp pain above the heel. A gap is palpable in the tendon although the appearance may be normal with the swelling associated. Treatment is usually repair and often the plantaris tendon can be used as a suture material. A cast is applied with the foot in equinus, or pointing downwards, and is kept in place for six weeks. Physiotherapy is necessary afterwards to restore function and strength to the calf.

    Conservative treatment can produce a reasonable result, but recurrence is more common.

2. **Biceps Tendon**

    This is commonly in the long head of biceps which passes through the shoulder and a characteristic lump appears in the upper arm on stressing the muscle. Pain may be felt prior to this due to inflammation of the tendon known as tendonitis. This is the author's right arm.

    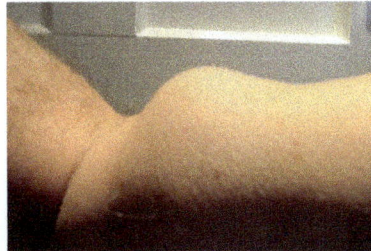

    (*There is a spelling mistake which persists in the orthopaedic literature in which inflammation of tendons is called tendinitis. A book has even been written about it, but just because it sounds like it does not mean to say it should be spelt like it; and we do not call a below knee plaster a baloney plaster for example*).

    Repair is not usually necessary as the other half of the bicep becomes stronger to compensate. It is very common in older men.

Notes:

DISORDERS OF THE UPPER LIMB

1. Frozen Shoulder (Capsulitis)

This is more common in women usually of middle age producing pain and stiffness, and later stiffness, and then gradual recovery. The pain is worse at night.

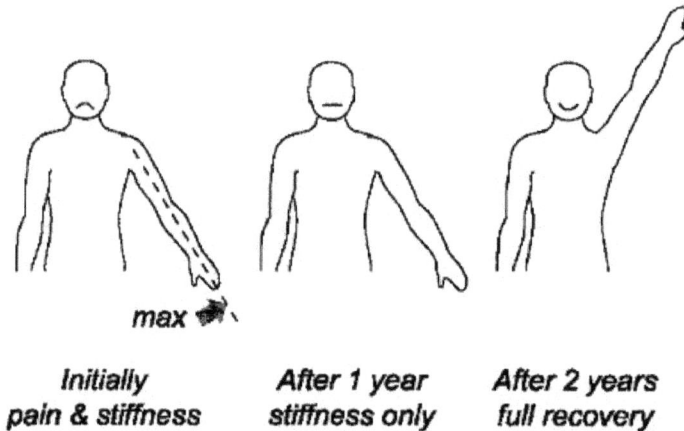

max

| Initially pain & stiffness | After 1 year stiffness only | After 2 years full recovery |

TREATMENT

Analgesics and anti-inflammatory tablets. Injection of local anaesthetic (LA) and steroids. Physiotherapy. Manipulation under anaesthetic (MUA). Arthroscopy. It usually resolves slowly over two years.

2. Rotator Cuff Lesion

This may be due to a partial or complete tear of the rotator cuff, usually the supraspinatus tendon. The rotator cuff is a group of muscles attached from the shoulder blade and passes to the upper end of the humerus. They pass beneath a bony ligamentous arch formed by the articulation between the distal clavicle and the distal spine of the scapula known as the acromion process at the AC or acromio-clavicular joint.

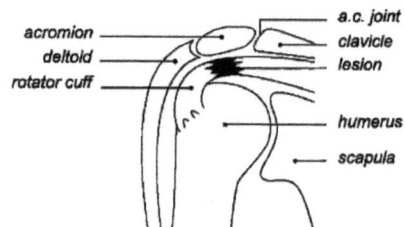

There is a painful arc of abduction, or inability to lift the arm from the side. This can be due to impingement.

Notes:

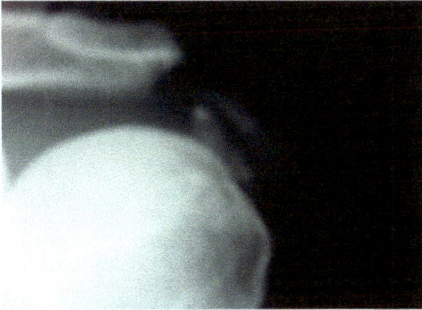

Calcification is sometime seen in the tendon as shown in the x-ray. An ultrasound scan or MRI scan can be an aid to diagnosis.

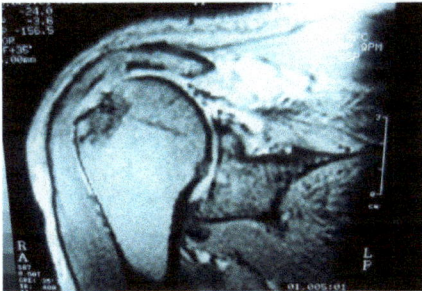

This is the author's right shoulder showing complete rupture with close proximity of the humeral head to the acromion.

TREATMENT

Conservative:

a) Analgesics and anti-inflammatories
b) Injection of local anaesthetic and steroid into the subacromial bursa, but usually no more than on three occasions
c) Physiotherapy in the form of ultrasound. Hydrotherapy, a TENS machine, and acupuncture may help.
d) Exercises such as swimming can produce strength in the deltoid to compensate although overhead activities are usually difficult unless surgical intervention takes place.

Surgical:

Surgery is indicated if there has been failure of relief from symptoms by conservative means and where a large tear has been demonstrated by ultrasound scanning. It is usually by arthroscopy and repair, together with subacromial decompression, and often excision of the distal end of the clavicle creating a fibrous arthroplasty at the acromio-clavicular joint. Reconstruction is occasionally needed when one can take the latissimus dorsi and transfer this muscle from the humerus to the great tuberosity.

Recovery:

Recovery often takes up to three months and physiotherapy is needed to assist.

3. **Lateral Epicondylitis ('tennis elbow'),** and

4. **Medial Epicondylitis ('golfer's elbow')**

Both are due to an irritation of the extensor and flexor muscle origins, although uncommon in either tennis players or golfers!

TREATMENT
Conservative:
Strapping, topical and systemic anti-inflammatories, injection LA and steroids, physiotherapy.

Surgical:
Release tendon and resuture.

5. **Repetitive Strain Injury (RSI)**
It is also known as WRULD (Work Related Upper Limb Disorder). Both are more a descriptive term than a diagnosis. It produces a painful forearm quite often in somewhat emotional young women, and often involving compensation. Therefore, it is often not believed, but is real to the individual.

It is interesting that it is uncommon in pianists or violinists who practice every day.

TREATMENT
Wrist supports. Change of work environment.

6. **De Quervain's Tenosynovitis**
This is an inflammation of the extensor tendons at the wrist producing swelling and crepitus. Named for **Fritz de Quervain**, 1868-1940, who was a general surgeon in Berne, also responsible for the introduction of iodised table salt used in the treatment of goitre.

TREATMENT
a) Topical and systemic anti-inflammatory tablets
b) Injection of local anaesthetic and steroid
c) Sometimes release of the tendon sheath

Notes:

7. Carpal Tunnel

This is a condition where there is compression of the median nerve at the wrist where it passes through the carpal tunnel together with the tendons that flex the fingers. It is common in middle-aged females and affects the thumb, index, and middle fingers particularly at night. The patient is often woken up at 2 or 3 o'clock in the morning and shakes the hand. This is a classic description for the condition. It can be confirmed by nerve conduction studies or EMG.

TREATMENT
Conservative:
Injection of local anaesthetic and steroid and a wrist splint with the hand in extension, to be worn at night.

Surgical:
Release of the flexor retinaculum at the wrist.

8. Trigger Finger

This is a condition where there is swelling in the flexor tendon in the palm producing a "catch" or jerk as the finger is bent and straightened. It can be seen in infants with a locked thumb.

TREATMENT
Percutaneous or open division of the palmar pulley.

9. Dupuytren's Contracture

This is named after **Baron Guillaume Dupuytren**, 1777-1835, born in poverty who rose to be a leading surgeon in France and Baron of the Empire.

It is due to thickening and fibrosis of the palmar fascia in the hand, mainly affecting the little and ring fingers which are slowly pulled into the palm.

Note the dimples in the palm, and the bent little finger.

Nodules are felt. It can occur in the feet.

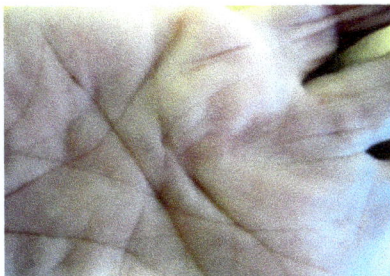

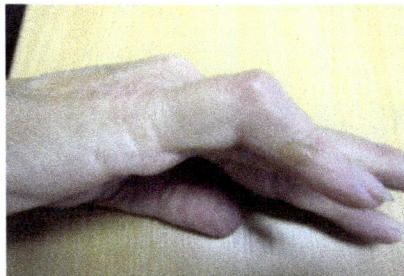

....

Notes:

Excision usually results in cure and if left too late it is difficult to sometimes get the finger out straight again without Z-plasty to the skin and sometimes there is permanent contracture of the MCP (metacarpal phalangeal) or PIP (proximal interphalangeal) joints.

10. Ulnar Nerve Compression

This commonly occurs at the elbow where the nerve passes behind the medical epicondyle, and less commonly through Guyon's canal at the wrist (**Felix Guyon**, 1831-1920).

Numbness of the little and the adjacent side of the ring finger and weakness of the small muscle of the hand (interossei) that help spread the fingers and bring them together. Diagnosis is confirmed by nerve conduction studies or EMG.

TREATMENT

Depending on the severity, release of the nerve or transposition to the ventral aspect of the elbow.

HAND INJURIES

They are important as we are the only animal on the planet able to pick up a pin from the table with our fingers and thumb.

The principles of treatment are:
- to assess the damage,
- to fix fractures, usually internally,
- to repair vessels and nerves.

Elevation and cold packs or ice are used to prevent swelling and it is most important to maintain and restore function with exercise as soon as possible.

Notes:

DISORDERS OF THE KNEE

1. Meniscal Lesions

Tears

The menisci in the knee are triangular in cross section and semilunar in shape. They are made of fibrocartilage.

The medial meniscus is damaged more commonly than the lateral, and in males more than females. It is common in footballers due to planting of the foot and twisting the body with the leg fixed, twisting the knee.

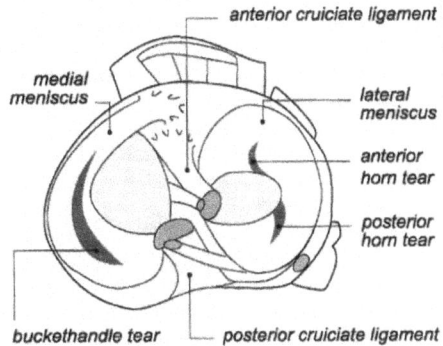

Cross-section of knee

anterior cruiciate ligament
medial meniscus
lateral meniscus
anterior horn tear
posterior horn tear
buckethandle tear
posterior cruiciate ligament

The cartilage is split by the overlying femoral condyle and there may be a bucket handle tear or a tear of the anterior or posterior horns.

Symptoms:
- There is usually a history of a twisting injury
- Pain and swelling
- Clicking or locking

Signs: A click or clunk on twisting the knee with the knee bent, first described by McMurray.

Tests: An x-ray is usually negative, but an MRI scan can show a tear.

TREATMENT:

Conservative: Exercises to strengthen the quadriceps or thigh muscle by swimming and cycling. Physiotherapy.

Surgical: Arthroscopic meniscectomy and occasionally repair of peripheral lesions to the capsule.

A late complication is arthritis after 20 years or more due to damage to the articular cartilage.

2. Anterior Knee Pain

This is common in young females often due to softening of the lining of the patella or kneecap otherwise called chondromalacia patella. The Female pelvis is wider relative to the male, so there is a slightly greater angle (Q angle) the femur makes with the tibia at the knee. This can alter the tension felt by the quadriceps muscle and its tendons as it passes to the tibia via the patella (a sesamoid bone nature places within tendons such as at the thumb and big toe and sometimes behind the knee). The patella slides in a shallow grove on the distal femur when the knee is bent.

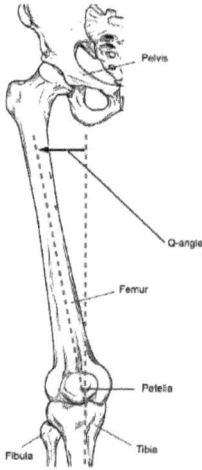

TREATMENT:
Conservative:
- Restrict sporting activities. Physiotherapy.
- Anti-inflammatory tablets.

Surgery: May involve realigning the patellar tendon. Shaving the patella by arthroscopy.

3. Cruciate Ligament Injuries
Rupture of the anterior cruciate (ACL) is common and of the posterior (PCL) uncommon, and are often associated with a tear of the medial ligament.

Symptoms: Similar to meniscal lesions with a twisting injury.

Signs:
a) There is a positive drawer sign but beware the backward sag of the knee in a PCL tear
b) Positive Lachman's test where the leg is grasped firmly and moved relative to the thigh with the knee bent
c) A pivot shift test may be positive with a subluxation of the tibia with the knee bent

Tests: MRI

TREATMENT:
Conservative:
a) Quadriceps drill
b) Physiotherapy
c) Splintage

Surgical:
Repair if acute, although mostly late reconstruction is necessary using natural tendons such as the patella or semi-tendinosis, or synthetic material. Six months recovery is needed with physiotherapy.

Notes:

SPINAL DISORDERS

The spine consists of a series of vertebrae interspersed with discs and which moves at the facet joints. Movement is effected by the paravertebral muscles which extend from the base of the back to the base of the head. The posterior muscles are stronger than the anterior as the centre of gravity is in front of the spine and they are required to maintain the vertical posture.

Because the spine is angulated at 30° to the horizontal in the lateral plane, there is a forward curve in the lower back called a **lordosis**, a backward curve in the thoracic spine called a **kyphosis**, and a forward curve in the neck called a **lordosis** to keep the head over the feet. The spine is numbered from the head down and is divided into sections:

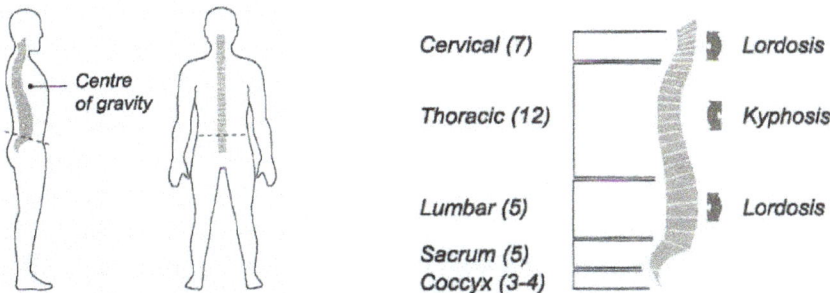

The head is quite heavy weighing 1.5–2kg and is supported on a relatively slender column of bone.

Most movement occurs in the neck and lower back, as the thoracic spine is relatively stiff to allow the ribs to move.

There is very little movement at each individual facet joint and the spine is strengthened by anterior and posterior longitudinal ligaments. There are ligaments between the spinous processes called the interspinous ligaments. With the combined movement most of us can bend over to touch our toes, although in my case they should be on my knees.

The disc is made up of a central nucleus surrounded by an outer laminated annulus fibrosis. It is similar to a rubber doughnut filled with thick jelly. It gives resilience to the spine. The annulus is thicker in front than behind, and if it becomes worn or is put under abnormal stress, the nucleus may prolapse (bulge through) usually posteriorly.

Notes:

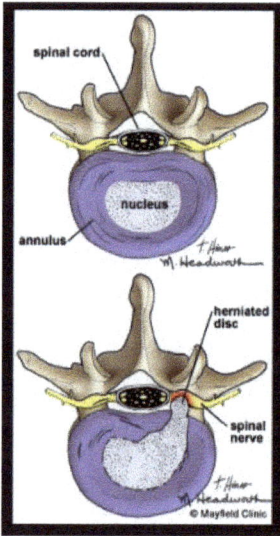

Pressure on the dura enclosing the spinal cord produces backache and pressure on the nerve root produces sciatica.

Most backaches, however, are due to stresses and strains in the soft tissues and are probably due to the fact that we are walking around on two legs on a high gravity planet with a spine that is not properly adapted to the upright posture.

Recovery occurs with exercise, physiotherapy and anti-inflammatory drugs.

Degeneration of the discs is common. It commences in the 20s such that by the 60s, nearly everybody has some degeneration in the discs, whether or not they have symptoms. It is commonly seen at C5/6 and C6/7 and L4/5 and L5/S1.

Images: Coronal view above, sagittal below

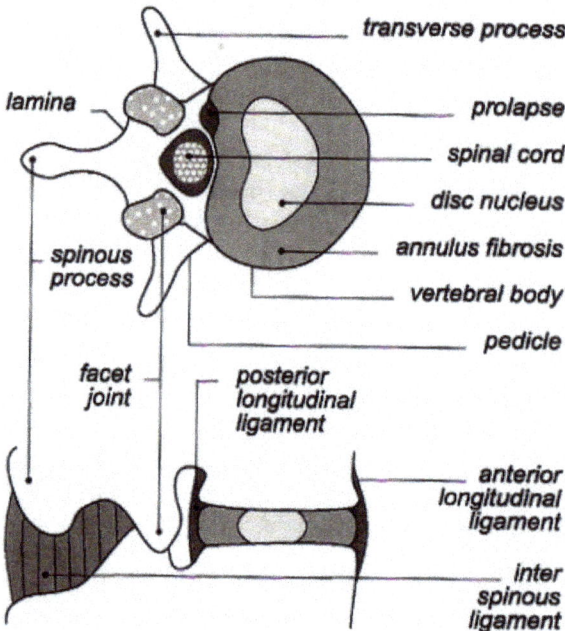

Notes:

ACUTE DISC PROLAPSE

This may be due to a blow to the head, sudden movement, heavy lifting or bending.

Symptoms:

- CS: neck pain and pain radiating down the arm known as brachialgia (armatica – author's term), or
- LS: low back pain and pain radiating down the leg known as sciatica.

Signs:

- Restricted movement
- Restricted straight leg raise (SLR)
- Muscle weakness
- Altered reflexes
- Altered sensation and paraesthesia may occur, usually along the dermatomes as shown.

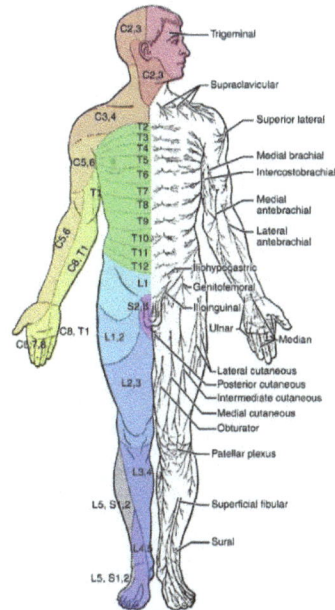

Tests: Plain x-ray shows loss of lordosis in the neck or back. CT scan. Discogram where dye is injected into the disc itself reproducing symptoms. MRI is the most helpful.

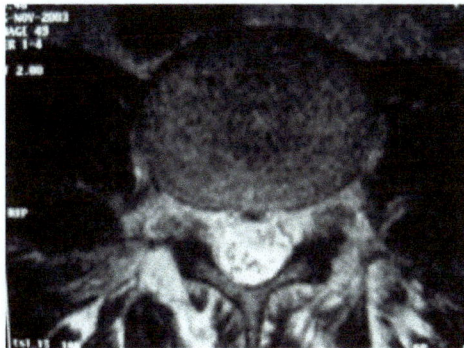
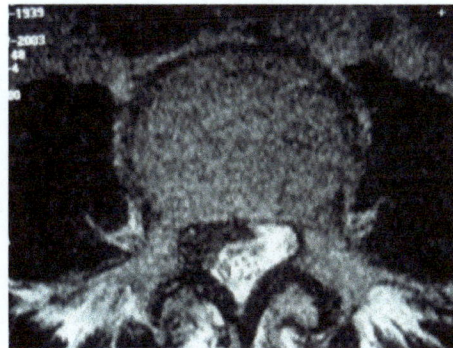

Normal   Prolapse

Notes:

This shows the author's L3/4 disc prolapse with compression of the L4 nerve root and numbness in the dermatome shown and weakness of the quadriceps, loss of the knee jerk and a normal disc for comparison.

Note the very narrow space at L5/S1 (previous disc resection) and old fracture L1.

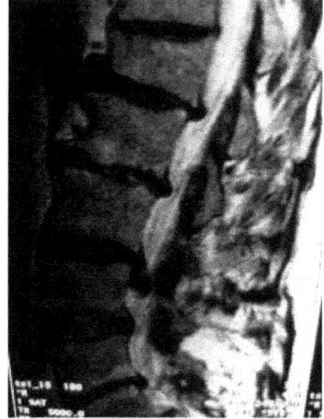

TREATMENT
Most patients recover without surgery (as did the author, on one occasion (L3/4), requiring surgery on another (L5/S1)).

Conservative:
- Rest: Bed rest for seven to ten days is often helpful with or without traction
- Drugs: Analgesics such as paracetamol or paracetamol mixed with codeine. I have noticed an increasing tendency for the use of tramadol, or oxycontin, which are opiate analgesics and more likely to produce addiction. Anti-inflammatory tablets provided they do not have side effects upsetting the stomach or provided the patient does not have asthma. Antispasmodics or muscle relaxants, such as diazepam or amitriptyline, may be helpful in the first two to three weeks.
- Local splintage with a collar or corset or brace
- The most important is an exercise programme such as swimming or cycling and walking without loading the spine. And:
    - Physiotherapy
    - Chiropractic
    - Osteopathy
    - Acupuncture
    - Epidural injections
    - Facet joint injections

In chronic cases the use of a pain clinic, and possible insertion of a stimulator.

Surgical:
Surgical treatment is indicated:
a) If the patient has bladder symptoms, urgent decompression of the spinal cord is necessary, as there may be an underlying cauda equina syndrome
b) If there has been failure of conservative treatment
c) There are positive neurological signs
d) A positive lesion seen on MRI scan

The surgical options are:

a) Foraminotomy

b) Laminectomy and discectomy with the aid of an operating microscope

c) Disc replacement is now used in some situations

d) Spinal fusion if the spine is unstable

CHRONIC/RECURRENT

This is most commonly seen in the low back and is known as the Low Back Syndrome.

Cause: Degenerate discs

Facet joint degeneration

Post traumatic scarring

One should consider alternative pathology such as a rectal carcinoma invading the sacrum or an abdominal aortic aneurysm

Symptoms: The pain is usually constant of a deep nagging nature. Radiation if the nerve root is involved.

Signs: Reduced movement is noted; in the neck one has to turn the body to reverse the car or use the wing mirrors, and in the low back difficulty in bending to put on socks is often noticed.

Tests:

*   X-ray: reduced disc space is noted with osteophyte formation or lipping. Facet joint narrowing.
*   MRI: dehydration in the discs, osteophytes, facet joint arthritis. May show spinal stenosis (narrowing of the canal).

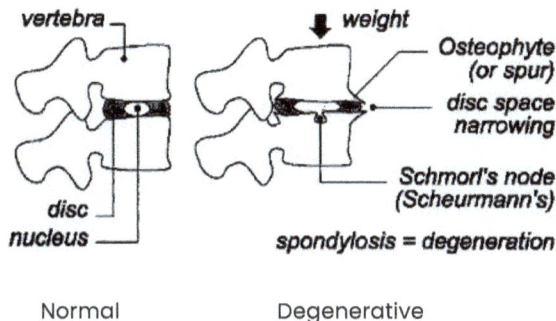

Normal   Degenerative

Notes:

TREATMENT

The two most important aspects of treatment are weight reduction and exercise. Stopping smoking is important as it has been shown that smoking affects the hydration of the disc with alteration of the vertebral end plate blood flow. A similar regime to the acute disc prolapse is recommended.

Surgery: Is indicated if there has been failure of conservative treatment, and may involve:

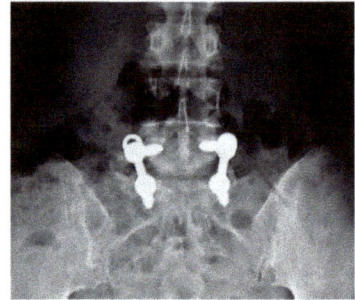

- Decompression
- Laminectomy
- Spinal fusion

Where compensation is involved, there is often a conscious or even an unconscious desire for gain and there are varying distinguishing signs that can be used to recognise patients who are not entirely genuine. Waddell described these some years ago although they were recognised prior to his article.

Signs:

- Restricted flexion of lumbar spine on standing but normal flexion on sitting up from the lying position
- Restricted SLR but can sit up with legs extended (equivalent to SLR 90°). "Cogwheel" flexion of hips when bending knees. Diminished sensation over the whole limb (glove and stocking) or even the whole side of the body.

Notes:

AMPUTATIONS

Removal of part of the body

Indications:

1. Dead limb – gangrene from arteriosclerosis or severe trauma
2. Lethal limb – may kill patient e.g., severe sepsis, malignant tumour
3. Nuisance – too frail, stiff, or deformed

Stump may be:

a) End bearing (weight through end of stump) e.g., through knee amputation. NB scar proximal
b) Non-end bearing (weight through soft tissues not end of stump) e.g., below knee amputation. Fish mouth scar.

Site of election:

Above knee   (AK) – 25cm below great trochanter

Below knee   (BK) – 12cm below tibial tubercle

Above elbow   (AE) – 20cm below tip of acromion

Below elbow   (BE) – 17cm below tip of olecranon

Technique:

1. Divide muscles, vessels (ligature), nerves (proximal), bone (bevel end).
2. Keep sufficient soft tissue – avoid bony adherence.
3. Important to bandage the stump to provide the best stump.

Professor Munjed al Muderis, 1972-, in Sydney, has developed 'Osteosynthesis' where an hydroxy-apatite coated titanium rod is inserted into the long bone in a limb, with 3-4cm protruding from the stump to which a prothesis or artificial limb can be attached with the aid of an Allen screw.

Before anaesthesia surgeons had to be very fast, especially in the European wars and a surgeon could amputate a leg in a minute. The patients often survived. Remember Long John Silver in "Treasure Island" with his wooden leg or Captain Ahab in "Moby Dick".

To fit an artificial limb:
- Immediate pylon
- Delayed fitting

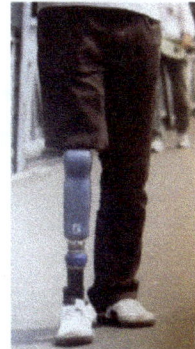

Notes:

Modern prostheses are very lifelike. The development of motors may enable some movement. New technology is enabling impulses sent by the patient's nerves to motors in the upper limb prostheses to invoke hand movement.

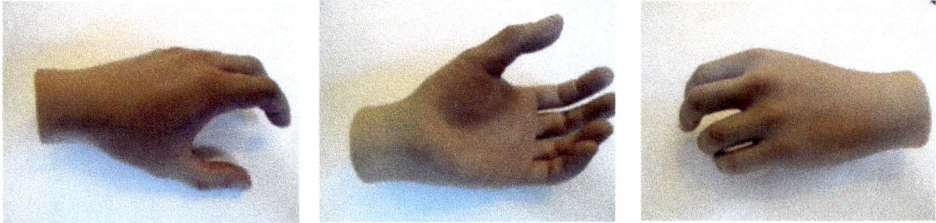

Below elbow amputation may be treated by separation of radius and ulna to give a pincer (Krukenberg operation, **Friedrich Kruckenberg**, 1871–1946).

This patient was treated by **Dr Ronald J Garst,** 1926–2009, in Bangladesh after the War of Independence in 1971.

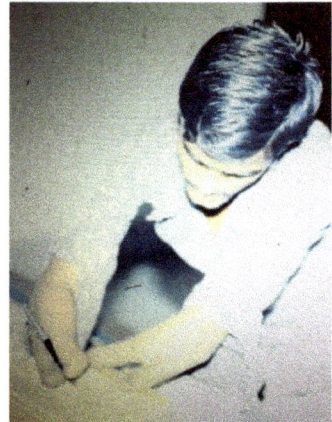

Complications:
1. Haemorrhage – leave tourniquet on the end of the bed
2. Skin problems with stump (scar too tight) – revise
3. Stump neuroma – excise more proximally.
4. Phantom limb – difficult to treat

Notes:

PART FOUR:

Neoplasia

Definition:

Mass of new tissue which persists and grows independently of its surrounding structures. Often called tumours which means a swelling.

BENIGN

Remains local, suffix –oma. Produces symptoms by pressure on surrounding tissue.

Bone – Osteoma

a) Ivory – lump on skull bones

b) Osteoid – central lucent core. Intense night pain relieved by aspirin. Often mid-shin.

Treatment: Excision

c) Cancellous

Cartilage – Chondroma

a) Enchondroma, inside bone, may cause pathological fracture

b) Ecchondroma, outside bone

Bone and cartilage – Osteochondroma

Bone capped with cartilage – Exostosis.

a) Single – usually ends of long bones – points away from growth plate

b) Multiple – diaphyseal aclasis – inherited. 5% become malignant

Fibrous tissue – Fibroma

Fibrous cortical defect. Fibrous dysplasia. These rarely cause symptoms and show as defects on x-ray with cyst formation or sclerosis.

Aneurysmal bone cyst

End of long bones – expansile – symptoms from pressure.

Unicameral bone cyst

Children – ends of long bones (common-humerus).

May present with pathological fracture due to enlarged bone and thin cortex.

Treatment for both: Curette and bone graft

Haemangioma

Rare – spine – backache – striated appearance on x-ray.

Treatment: Radiotherapy

Notes:

INTERMEDIATE

Locally invasive.

Osteoclastoma

Giant cell tumour. Swelling at end of long bone usually in young adults, often painful.

Treatment: Curette and bone graft

Radiotherapy

MALIGNANT

Invade surrounding tissue and metastasise via bloodstream and lymphatics to produce secondary deposits (metatases).

Primary tumours

Rare.

Osteosarcoma

Young, 10-20 years old. 5% Paget's disease, often end of long bones. Pain, swelling. Early spread by blood stream.

X-ray: Codman's triangle (**Ernest Codman,** 1869-1940), sun ray appearance on x-ray due to periosteal elevation and bone formation.

Treatment: Amputation, radiotherapy, chemotherapy

65-75% 5-year survival rate, depending on spread

Chondrosarcoma

Adults' flat bones (scapula, pelvis) ends long bone metastasise late.

Treatment: Resection

Fibrosarcoma

Often end femur, proximal tibia. Pain, swelling.

Treatment: Amputate

Ewing's Tumour (James Ewing, 1866-1943)

10-20 years old, mid shaft commonly tibia. Onion skin appearance on x-ray due to new bone formation as periosteum is lifted.

Treatment: Excise (amputate) chemotherapy

Notes:

Multiple Myeloma

Middle aged, pain, x-ray punched out "holes" in bones. Bence-Jones protein in urine. CRAB (increased **C**alcium levels in blood, **R**enal dysfunction, **A**naemia, **B**one pain).

Treatment:

Local radiotherapy if practicable, induction chemotherapy, proteasome inhibitor (bortezomib), dexamethasone, immunotherapy.

Leukaemia

Ache in bones, fatigue (anaemia).

Treatment: Chemotherapy

Secondary tumours (metastases)

These are the most common form of bone tumours, and although carcinoma spreads mainly via the lymphatics, blood stream spread to multiple sites in bones is common in carcinoma of the:

a) Breast

b) Prostate

c) Lung

d) Kidney

e) Thyroid

Bone pain, pathological fractures

Treatment: Internally fix

CARE OF THE DYING PATIENT

1. Analgesia – do not withhold opiates
2. Good nursing – soft pillows and sheets, TLC
3. Do not resuscitate – death is a release

Notes:

TUMOURS AND CYSTS OF SOFT TISSUES

Ganglion
Common in wrist – jelly, but feels hard.
Treatment: Aspirate or excise

Semimembranosus Cyst
Behind knee – common in young boys, trans-illuminates.
Treatment: Excise

Baker's Cyst (William Baker, 1838-1896)
Behind knee synovial swelling associated arthritis.
Treatment: None

Lipoma
Soft swelling in the subcutaneous tissues.
Treatment: Reassure or excise

Fibroma
Firmer lump.

Neurofibromatosis
Multiple lumps in the skin, brown stains (café au lait), giant limbs (elephantiasis).

Neuroma
a) Amputation – pain
Treatment: Excise more proximally

b) Morton's (Thomas Morton, 1835-1903) – pain, metatarsalgia, sole of foot usually 3-4 cleft between metatarsal heads
Treatment: Metatarsal insoles, excise

Bursitis
Inflammatory swelling of bursa (like a small hot water bottle) that nature places over bony prominences.
a) Olecranon – drinker's elbow
b) Knee – housemaid's knee (pre-patellar bursitis)
Treatment: Anti-inflammatory drugs, injection of local anaesthetic and steroid, excise.

Notes:

Plantar fasciitis

Inflammatory reaction of attachment of plantar fascia to inferior surface of calcaneus (os calcis or heel bone) and may produce a spur on lateral x-ray.

Treatment: Silicone heel cups, injection of local anaesthetic and steroid, excise.

Heberden's nodes (**William Heberden,** 1710-1801)

Small, painless, hard swellings at the distal inter-phalangeal (DIP) joints of the fingers.

Treatment. None

Bouchard's nodes (**Charles-Joseph Bouchard,** 1837-1915)

Similar to Heberden's nodes but associated with the proximal inter-phalangeal (PIP) joints of the fingers but are less frequently seen.

Treatment. None

Notes:

PART FIVE:

Degenerative Conditions

Synovial joints are affected by various disease processes: rheumatoid arthritis, osteoarthritis, gouty arthritis, anklylosing spondylitis, hallux rigidus, and hallux valgus. Pagets is a disease of bone.

RHEUMATOID ARTHRITIS

1.   Aetiology: unknown, possibly auto-immune
2.   20-40 yrs. Female: male, 3:1
3.   Commences in the synovium: inflamed (synovitis), thickened (pannus), rheumatoid nodule, effusion
4.   Gradually destroys articular cartilage – direct action
5.   Ligaments become stretched, lax – deformity
6.   Tendon sheaths affected – tendons may rupture (dropped fingers)
7.   Relapses and remissions occur – may burn out

Symptoms:
• Pain, one joint or several (polyarthritis)
• Malaise
• Stiffness

Signs:
• Joints swollen, signs of inflammation
• Commonly small joints of the hands
• Synovial swelling and rheumatoid nodules
• Late: deformity in the hands – MCP joints – Ulnar drift, dropped fingers (ruptured extensor tendons). IP joints Boutonniere, swan neck. Feet – claw toes, bunions, and hallux valgus

Tests:
• Blood:
  • Raised ESR
  • Positive Rose Waaler and latex (75%)
  • Positive C reactive protein

• X-rays:
  • Osteoporosis, erosion
  • Joint space narrowing
  • Deformity

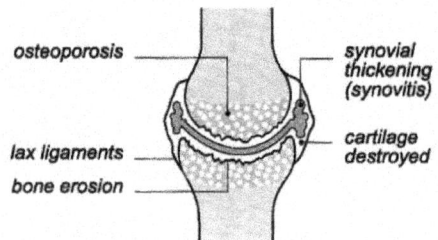

Notes:

TREATMENT:

General:

Drugs:

a) Analgesics e.g., aspirin (also NSAIDs)

b) NSAIDs (non-steroidal anti-inflammatory drugs) inhibit cyclo-oxygenase (COX) the enzyme producing prostaglandins but also produces side effects such as gastric mucosal irritation

c) Anti-arthritic, gold, chloroquine

d) Suppressant, steroids e.g., prednisolone – long term side effects: Cushing's syndrome (thin skin with increased capillary fragility), bruises, osteoporosis, avascular necrosis (hip joint), obesity (moon face, buffalo hump)

e) TNF – alpha blockers (tumour necrosis factor) e.g., etanercept, infliximab

f) Methotrexate

Local:

a) Splintage – physiotherapy

b) Synovectomy

c) Salvage – arthroplasty

Notes:

OSTEOARTHRITIS (OA)

Degeneration in a joint. A better term is osteoarthrosis but through usage osteoarthritis is accepted. Degeneration commences in the articular cartilage and can be likened to the wearing out of a carpet. Firstly, there is loss of the sheen (chondromalacia), then there is gradually loss of the fibre (fibrillation), wear is down to the under-felt (ulceration), and finally through to the floorboards (bare bone).

It is a gradually progressive condition and is common in the weight-bearing joints and also the joints of the spine.

It is less commonly seen in the upper limb than in the lower limb and surprisingly rare in the ankle although this is the joint most frequently injured by sprains and fractures.

Cause and progression:

1. Damage to articular cartilage – by trauma, faulty stresses, vascular problems, irritants (e.g., gout) producing chondromalacia – softening and fibrillation of cartilage

2. Damage to synovial lining – fibrosis of capsule, stretching and causes pain, gradually restricting movement

3. Damage to bone – subchondral sclerosis, osteophyte formation, cysts Lipping

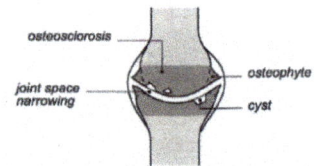

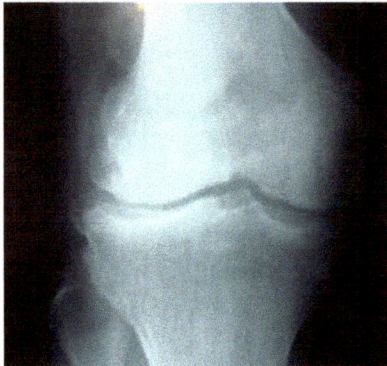

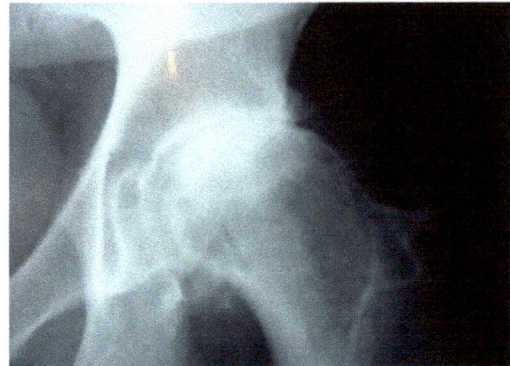

Note the changes in the lateral compartment of the knee, and in the hip.

Notes:

Symptoms:
- Pain
- Deformity
- Loss of function
- Limp
- Swelling

Signs:
- Decreased range of movement
- Crepitus – grating on movement
- Limping – if in joints of the lower limb
- Heberden's nodes in fingers

Tests:
- X-ray: Loss of joint space
- Sclerosis
- Lipping or osteophyte formation
- Cysts

Causes of a limp from hip problems throughout life:
- 0-3: DDH
- 3-5: TB, Transient synovitis (irritable hip)
- 5-10: Perthe's
- 0-15: Slipped epiphysis
- 15-35: Trauma
- 35-50: OA secondary to preceding conditions
- 50+: Primary OA

TREATMENT:
General:
- Rest – reduce activity, use walking stick
- Diet – reduce weight
- Drugs – analgesics, anti-inflammatories (NSAIDs), glucosamine, chondroitin, hyaluronic acid

Conservative:
a) Physiotherapy – ultrasound, exercises, shortwave diathermy, massage, heat
b) Manipulation

Notes:

c) Built-up shoe

d) Injections into joint – hyaluronate or steroids

e) Arthroscopy and wash out

Surgical:

Osteotomy, arthroplasty, arthrodesis.

- Osteotomy – surgical fracture to alter stresses through joint. Internal or external fixation
- Arthroplasty – refashion a joint
  1. Excision arthroplasty – create a gap to fill with scar tissue by removing part of the bone ends
  2. Replace one or both end of the bone with a prosthesis e.g., THR (total hip replacement), TKR (total knee replacement)
  3. Cartilage grafting or possibly stem cell replacement in the future

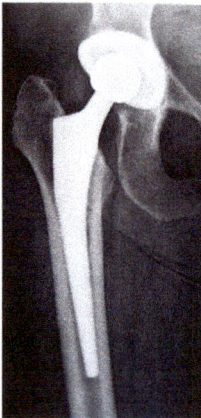

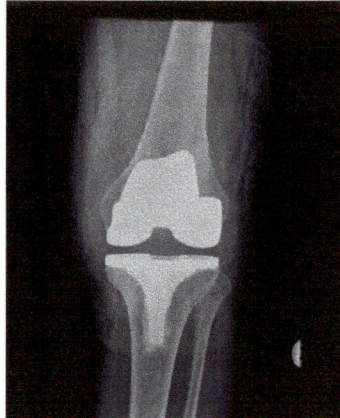

- Arthrodesis – this is fusion of the bone ends. The trade is loss of pain for loss of movement. Failure to fuse results in a pseudarthrosis (false joint)

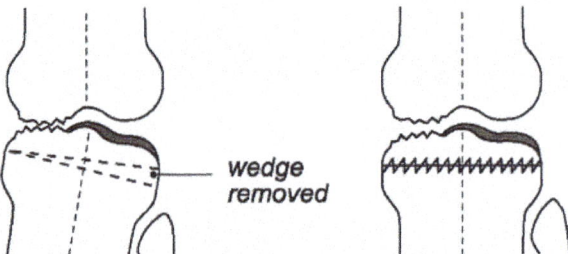

Above: Osteotomy surgical treatment   Above: Author's ankle

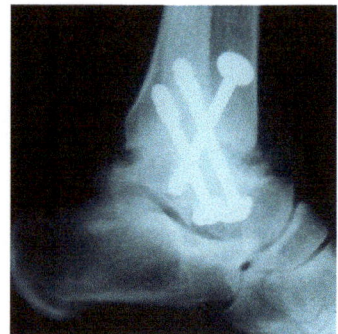

Complications:

General:

1. Blood loss – shock.
    Treatment: Blood replacement, may need to re-operate to find bleeding source.

2. Deep vein thrombosis/pulmonary embolism
    Prevent: Low molecular weight heparin/aspirin, elastic stockings (TED – thrombo-embolic disease), calf compression or foot compression, pumps in theatre and after surgery
    Symptoms: Calf pain, chest pain
    Signs: Calf tenderness, pleural rub
    Tests: Doppler, Venogram, VQ lung scan
    Treatment: Anticoagulants – Heparin ten days, Warfarin three months

Local:

1. Dislocation
    Prevent: Abduction pillows in hip replacements
    Treatment: Relocate – may need to re-operate and change alignment (usually socket).

2. Infection
    Prevent: Preoperative, operative and postoperative broad-spectrum antibiotics
    Treatment: Antibiotics – drain. May need exchange prosthesis – difficult. High risk of failure

3. Loosening
    Late complication, usually after ten years
    Prevent: Compression cementing technique, hydroxyapatite coated prostheses in uncemented procedures
    Treatment: Revision difficult – operation twice as long as primary procedure.
    May need to convert to excision arthroplasty (**G. R. Girdlestone,** 1881-1950).

Notes:

GOUT

This is caused by an increased uric acid level in the blood that produces crystals in the synovium and leads to inflammation. Cartilage may be damaged and leads to arthritis.

Note the white deposits of uric acid crystals in the knee.

It is commonly seen in the small joints of the foot (especially the great toe) and in the hand., causing pain and loss of function.

TREATMENT:

General:

Drugs – anti-inflammatory; allopurinol – decreased formation uric acid, probenecid – increased excretion by kidney.

Surgical: As for osteoarthritis.

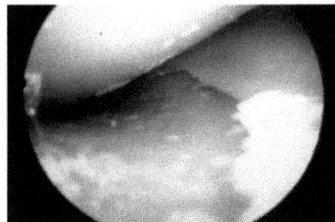

ANKYLOSING SPONDYLITIS

An inflammatory condition of the spine: progressive, males > females. Commences usually in the sacroiliac joints.

Symptoms: Pain, aching more than acute. Stiffness.

Signs: Local tenderness. Decreased movement, loss of extension leading to a bent forward position.

Tests:

- Blood – HLA antigen positive
- X-ray – sclerosis and bone loss in the sacroiliac joints. Bone formation in the apophyseal or facet joints of the spine, ossification of the discs leading to bamboo spine.

TREATMENT:

Conservative:

- Anti-inflammatory drugs
- Physiotherapy – emphasis on exercise and posture

Surgical:

- Osteotomy of the spine if the bent forward posture is greater than 45°

Notes:

HALLUX RIGIDUS, HALLUS VALGUS AND BUNIONS

Hallux rigidus is OA (osteoarthritis) of the metatarso-phalangeal (MTP) joint of the big toe and pressure from osteophytes. The joint is usually stiff.

Hallux valgus is an outer sideways deviation of the big toe, often associated with a medial or inner deviation of the metatarsal. An exostosis develops on the head of the metatarsal known as a bunion.

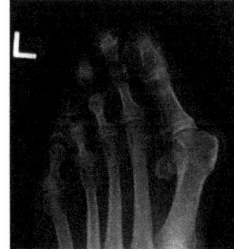

- **Symptoms:** Pain from pressure of shoes
- **Signs:** Deviated toe, prominent bunion. Reduced movement in the MTP joint in hallux rigidus with increased extension in the IP joint. Second toe often too long and forms a hammer toe with fixed flexion of PIP joint
- **Tests:** X-rays show medial deviation of the metatarsal and lateral deviation of the toe with an exostosis (bunion) on the medial side of the 1st metatarsal, or osteophytes and joint space narrowing in hallux rigidus.

TREATMENT:

Conservative: Relieve pressure by felt ring, hole in shoe, metatarsal bar.

Surgical:

a) Remove bunion – exostectomy

b) Osteotomy metatarsal or proximal phalanx

c) Arthroplasty - excision, Keller's (**William Keller,** 1874-1959), replacement (silastic or titanium)

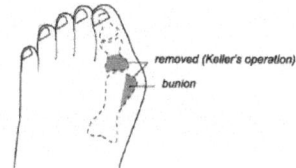

removed (Keller's operation)

bunion

d) Arthrodesis – fusion MTP joint +/- (PIP 2nd toe)

Notes:

PAGET'S DISEASE

Named after **Sir James Paget**, 1814-1899, one of the great Victorians.

Male > female 50-70 age group.

Cause unknown. Thickening of bone with osteoblastic and clastic activity – spongy soft bone. 5% malignant change.

Symptoms: Pain.

Signs: Deformity, Increasing hat size, bent bones, stress fractures.

Tests: X-ray – mixed osteoporotic and blastic activity.

TREATMENT:

Conservative:

Drugs – Analgesics, fluoride, bisphosphonates.

Surgical:

- Osteotomy
- Intramedullary rods for stress fractures in long bone

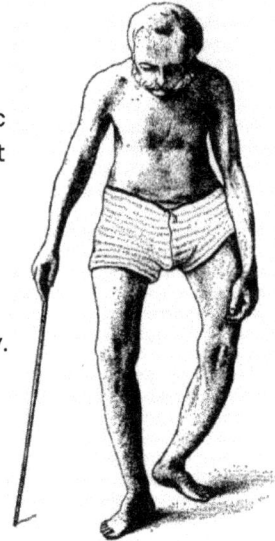

Paget's Disease

Notes:

PART SIX:

Metabolic, Endocrine, Immunological

VITAMIN DEFICIENCY

Vitamin D

Rickets – soft bones especially distal tibia. Prevent by exposure to sunlight to stimulate melanoblasts and treat with vitamin supplement.

Vitamin C

Scurvy – subperiosteal haemorrhage. Pain, loose teeth, bleeding, death.

TREATMENT: Fresh fruit, vitamin supplement (British sailors in the 18th Century were known as 'Limeys' as they were provided with limes to prevent scurvy on long voyages).

ACROMEGALY

This is an endocrine disorder with excessive growth hormone excreted by the pituitary gland leading to gigantism. There is the skeleton of the Irish Giant standing 2.25 metres tall in the Royal College of Surgeons Museum in London prepared by **John Hunter**, 1728-1793, (another of my heroes in Medicine), displayed next to the Sicilian dwarf of 55cm also from his collection.

OSTEOMALACIA

Loss of calcium from bone – malnutrition, post gastrectomy.

TREATMENT: Calcium, vitamin D.

OSTEOPOROSIS

Loss of calcium as absorption greater than formation leads to decreased quantity of bone. Pathological fractures common.

1. Postmenopausal
2. Disuse
3. Elderly
4. Dowager hump

TREATMENT: HRT (hormone replacement therapy), exercises (most important), no response to vitamin D, but use of Calcichew and Alendronate. Treat fractures as appropriate.

Notes:

COMPLEX REGIONAL PAIN SYNDROME

Previously called Reflex Sympathetic Dystrophy.

This is an altered vascular response, often to minor trauma, and leads to demineralisation of bone, changes in the skin and disabling pain which is difficult to treat. Spontaneous resolution can occur. Sympathectomy in some cases.

FIBROMYALGIA

Chronic pain syndrome felt in the muscles and joints, but diagnosis still somewhat in dispute.

Notes:

PART SEVEN:

Psychosomatic

Everyone has problems and sometimes people find relief from their problems through imaginary illnesses or gaining attention from real illnesses. The glass seems to be half empty rather than half full.

Placebo medication (no active ingredients) can provide relief in about 30% of cases, even with known diseases. Where a true psychotic state exists a diagnosis of conversion hysteria can be made. Treatment is extremely difficult. Even Psychiatrists find treating these patients hard.

The system of payment for injury may result in patients not wanting to get better from genuine injuries or feigning symptoms and signs (malingering), and the examining doctor for the Court has to be as objective as possible. The system of blame and claim seems to be becoming more and more prevalent, fuelled by lawyers. "I have been hurt and someone must pay for my pain and loss of amenity" is a common underlying, though often unexpressed, thought process.

With children, abuse must be suspected if a fracture occurs under the age of two with a doubtful history, and there are numerous examples of a child being returned to abusive parents because doctors, nurses and social workers do not suspect that some parents could mistreat their children.

We all have our own foibles and must be as objective and understanding as possible when dealing with patients.

Notes:

PART EIGHT:

Iatrogenic

Doctors are in a position where they can help many people return to health and most doctors enter the profession to do just that. However, sometimes mistakes happen, e.g., prescribing a drug where there is a known allergy, or an injection wrongly sited damaging a nerve for example. There is no guarantee in medicine, but an expectation that treatment will be successful.

Negligence is accepted where a doctor falls **below** the standard of care considered by his peers to be reasonable. Often it is the system at fault and not just the individual and when deficiencies in practice occur the whole approach must be examined.

When administering a drug or giving a blood transfusion it is always best to check the dose or blood label with a second person. Giving adult doses to children is a common mistake, or mistaking milligrams for micrograms. A doctor or patient should never be embarrassed about getting a second opinion, particularly if major surgery is involved.

Advice must be tempered with knowledge, and it is important to have a clear understanding of what treatment is to be given, before undertaking that treatment, and making sure consent is given on the basis of understanding. As one teacher said to me, "Know thy limitations", and I pass it on to you.

Notes:

PART NINE:

Summary

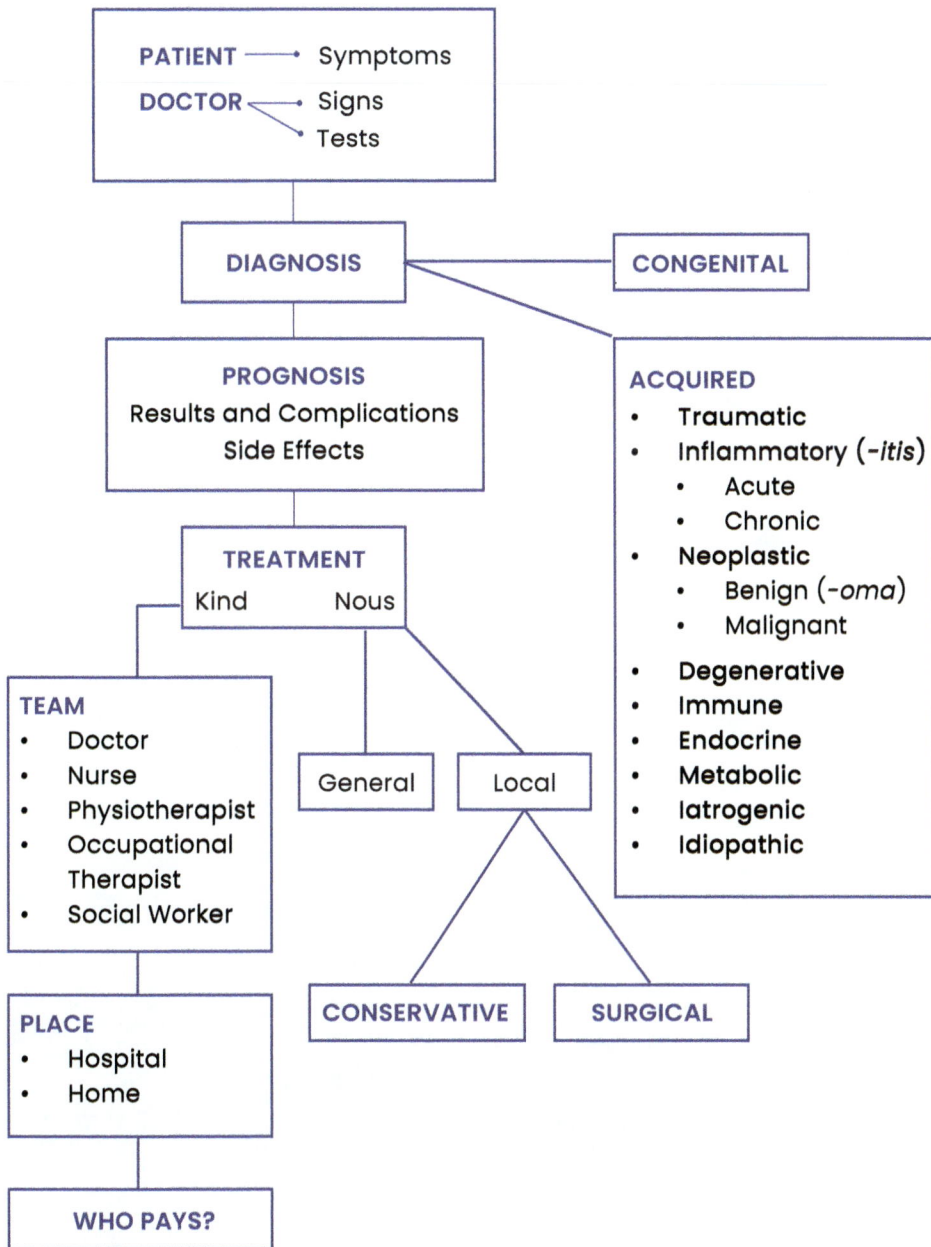

PATIENT ——• Symptoms

DOCTOR ——• Signs
           ——• Tests

DIAGNOSIS ———— **CONGENITAL**

PROGNOSIS
Results and Complications
Side Effects

ACQUIRED
- **Traumatic**
- **Inflammatory** (*-itis*)
  - Acute
  - Chronic
- **Neoplastic**
  - Benign (*-oma*)
  - Malignant
- **Degenerative**
- **Immune**
- **Endocrine**
- **Metabolic**
- **Iatrogenic**
- **Idiopathic**

TREATMENT
Kind   Nous

TEAM
- Doctor
- Nurse
- Physiotherapist
- Occupational Therapist
- Social Worker

General   Local

CONSERVATIVE   **SURGICAL**

PLACE
- Hospital
- Home

WHO PAYS?

Notes:

INDEX

A

B

C

M

N

O

P

APPENDIX

IMAGE ACKNOWLEDGMENTS

The author would like to thank the following for permission to reproduce their material. Every care has been taken to trace copyright holders but if there have been unintentional infringements or failure to acknowledge copyright holders accurately, then I apologise and will endeavour to make amends in future editions.

Cover, 1, 126: The Story of Orthopaedics by Mercer Rang;

5: Wellcome Collections CCA license, photo number L0004966 (https://wellcomecollection.org/works/hmteb4fd), originally from De Motu Cordis (1628);

6: Wikimedia Commons CCA-SA license, author Catherine Munro;

8, 9, 12: Dr Jennifer Philps;

10: Author unknown, public domain image (http://www.pdimages.com/web9.htm);

11, 24 (top), 26, 34 (top two), 39, 51, 52, 54, 58, 59, 60 (bottom), 61, 63 (top), 69, 73, 74, 79, 84 (top), 88 (top), 96, 101, 103, 104 (bottom), 107, 118, 120 (top), 122 (bottom left), 125 (bottom): Jo & Joe Design UK;

14 (top): Scientific Animations CCA-SA license (https://scientificanimations.com/ wiki-images);

14 (bottom two), 15 (top), 23, 28: The Atlas of the Human Body by P. Abrahams;

15 (bottom): Wikimedia Commons CCA license, artwork by Holly Fischer;

16: PLOS Biology, CCA license, authors Lars Chittka and Axel Brockmann (doi:10.1371/ journal.pbio.0030137);

18, 105 (top): Medical Gallery of Mikael Häggström 2014 (doi:10.15347/wjm/2014.008);

20: "OLI – Drawing Interaction of blood and lymphatic vessels – English labels" at AnatomyTOOL.org by Open Learning Initiative, CC BY-NC-SA license;

22: Concepts in Biology CCA-SA license (https://schoolbag.info/biology/concepts/94.html);

29: The Anatomical Drawings of Andreas Vesalius by J.B. de C.M. Saunders & C.D. O'Malley;

32: Wellcome Collections CCA license, image number 568245i;

87: Public domain image, Flickr image number 14783612943;

102: Openstax.org: Anatomy and Physiology CCA licence (http://cnx.org.content/col11496l/1.6, June 19, 2013);

104 (top): Mayfield Clinic, image created by Martha Headworth and Tonya Hines.

www.ingramcontent.com/pod-product-compliance
Lightning Source LLC
Chambersburg PA
CBHW051618030426
42334CB00030B/3248